PSYCHIATRY - THEORY, APPLICATIONS AND TREATMENTS

# TRICHOTILLOMANIA (HAIR PULLING DISORDER)

## CLINICAL CHARACTERISTICS, PSYCHOLOGICAL INTERVENTIONS AND EMOTIONAL EFFECTS

# PSYCHIATRY - THEORY, APPLICATIONS AND TREATMENTS

Additional books in this series can be found on Nova's website under the Series tab.

Additional e-books in this series can be found on Nova's website under the eBooks tab.

# DERMATOLOGY - LABORATORY AND CLINICAL RESEARCH

Additional books in this series can be found on Nova's website under the Series tab.

Additional e-books in this series can be found on Nova's website under the eBooks tab.

PSYCHIATRY - THEORY, APPLICATIONS AND TREATMENTS

# TRICHOTILLOMANIA (HAIR PULLING DISORDER)

## CLINICAL CHARACTERISTICS, PSYCHOLOGICAL INTERVENTIONS AND EMOTIONAL EFFECTS

KATLEIN FRANÇA
AND
MOHAMMAD JAFFERANY
EDITORS

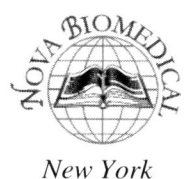

New York

Copyright © 2017 by Nova Science Publishers, Inc.

**All rights reserved.** No part of this book may be reproduced, stored in a retrieval system or transmitted in any form or by any means: electronic, electrostatic, magnetic, tape, mechanical photocopying, recording or otherwise without the written permission of the Publisher.

We have partnered with Copyright Clearance Center to make it easy for you to obtain permissions to reuse content from this publication. Simply navigate to this publication's page on Nova's website and locate the "Get Permission" button below the title description. This button is linked directly to the title's permission page on copyright.com. Alternatively, you can visit copyright.com and search by title, ISBN, or ISSN.

For further questions about using the service on copyright.com, please contact:
Copyright Clearance Center
Phone: +1-(978) 750-8400   Fax: +1-(978) 750-4470   E-mail: info@copyright.com.

### NOTICE TO THE READER

The Publisher has taken reasonable care in the preparation of this book, but makes no expressed or implied warranty of any kind and assumes no responsibility for any errors or omissions. No liability is assumed for incidental or consequential damages in connection with or arising out of information contained in this book. The Publisher shall not be liable for any special, consequential, or exemplary damages resulting, in whole or in part, from the readers' use of, or reliance upon, this material. Any parts of this book based on government reports are so indicated and copyright is claimed for those parts to the extent applicable to compilations of such works.

Independent verification should be sought for any data, advice or recommendations contained in this book. In addition, no responsibility is assumed by the publisher for any injury and/or damage to persons or property arising from any methods, products, instructions, ideas or otherwise contained in this publication.

This publication is designed to provide accurate and authoritative information with regard to the subject matter covered herein. It is sold with the clear understanding that the Publisher is not engaged in rendering legal or any other professional services. If legal or any other expert assistance is required, the services of a competent person should be sought. FROM A DECLARATION OF PARTICIPANTS JOINTLY ADOPTED BY A COMMITTEE OF THE AMERICAN BAR ASSOCIATION AND A COMMITTEE OF PUBLISHERS.

Additional color graphics may be available in the e-book version of this book.

### Library of Congress Cataloging-in-Publication Data

ISBN: 978-1-53610-854-5
Library of Congress Control Number: 2017930504

*Published by Nova Science Publishers, Inc. † New York*

*I dedicate this book to my father and mother, who have encouraged and guided me in my professional and personal evolution.*

*I dedicate this book to the rest of my beautiful Brazilian family. I am very fortunate to have you all in my life.*

*I dedicate this book to my patients, professors, mentors and friends. Thank you for this great journey.*

*Katlein França*

*I dedicate this book with love and affection to my both parents who are in Heaven. If it weren't for you, I am sure I wouldn't be who I am today. I love you both.*

*Mohammad Jafferany*

# Contents

| | | |
|---|---|---|
| **Foreword** | | ix |
| | *Jerry Shapiro* | |
| **Acknowledgments** | | xi |
| **About the Editors** | | xiii |
| **List of Contributors** | | xvii |
| **Chapter 1** | The History of Trichotillomania: The Bible, Shakespeare, and Other Curiosities<br>*Katlein França, Angela Y. Kim and Torello Lotti* | 1 |
| **Chapter 2** | Trichotillomania in Trichopsychodermatology<br>*Katlein França* | 11 |
| **Chapter 3** | Trichotillomania: Basic Concepts<br>*Mohammad Jafferany and Ferdnand C. Osuagwu* | 17 |
| **Chapter 4** | Dermatopathology and Trichotillomania<br>*Bárbara Roque Ferreira, José Pedro Reis and José Carlos Cardoso* | 35 |
| **Chapter 5** | Pharmacotherapy<br>*David Castillo, Clinton Enos, Katlein França and Torello Lotti* | 55 |
| **Chapter 6** | Non-Pharmacological Treatments for Trichotillomania<br>*Philip D. Shenefelt* | 75 |

| **Chapter 7** | Trichotillomania and the Emotion Regulation Hypothesis<br>*Erin E. Curley and Nancy J. Keuthen* | **85** |

**Index** **101**

# Foreword

Trichotillomania is a very complex and one of the most difficult problems to treat in our dermatologic clinics. One may consider it more of a psychiatric rather than a dermatologic disorder. However, the patient usually presents to the dermatologist and almost all dermatologists feel inadequate in confirming the diagnosis and in treating it adequately. This book is a very important addition to our "hair" libraries. It guides us in terms of confirmation of diagnosis and managing the problem. The concept of trichopsychodermatology is new term all dermatologists should become familiar with. This condition affects all age groups and is described well in the book. The chapters cover clinical features, dermatopathology, trichoscopic features, pharmacologic, non-pharmacological treatments, behavior therapy, and the concept of emotion regulation. The book is rich in photographs and figures that help explain the condition. Every hair clinic should have access to a book such as this to help provide a road map for the dermatologist and psychotherapist as to what to do and what can be done.

The Editors Drs. Katlein Franca and Mohammad Jafferany have put together a comprehensive book on this puzzling hair disorder and have compiled the most knowledgeable experts in the field to give their opinions on practical diagnosis and management plans. It is the first book of its kind and should be read by all dermatologists.

Jerry Shapiro, MD, FAAD
Professor
Disorders of the Scalp and Hair
The Robert O. Perelman Department of Dermatology
New York University School of Medicine, New York, New York

# ACKNOWLEDGMENTS

"If I have seen further it is by standing on the shoulders of giants"
(Isaac Newton)

We sincerely thank all the authors of this book, whose untiring efforts in writing chapters for this book have resulted in significant contribution in literature on trichotillomania. We highly appreciate their work. Without their research and contribution, the production of this book would not have been possible. Our patients with trichotillomania also inspired us to explore this condition and gave us a new perspective of the management of this neglected disease. We are also inspired with the work of Association for Psychoneurocutaneous Medicine of North America (APMNA), European Society of Dermatology and Psychiatry (ESDaP), Psychodermatology Group of the Brazilian Society of Dermatology, Japanese Society of Psychosomatic Medicine and UK Psychodermatology group. All these organizations, societies and groups have inspired us tremendously to edit a book on this important subject. We are also indebted to our families for their patience and support during the entire time we were working on writing and editing this book. We are also thankful to Nova Science Publishers for providing the opportunity to bring this book for the readership. It has been a pleasure working with them in this inspiring project.

*Katlein França, MD, PhD*
*Mohammad Jafferany, MD*

# ABOUT THE EDITORS

## KATLEIN FRANCA, MD, MSc, PhD

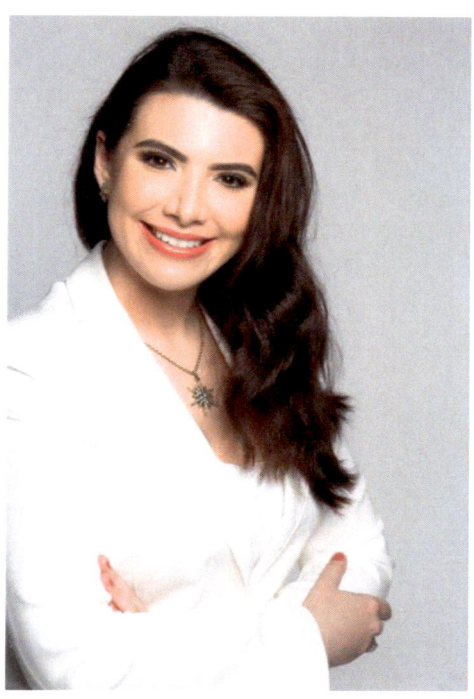

Dr. Katlein França is a dermatologist and PhD in Psychology. She is the President of the Association for Psychoneurocutaneous Medicine of North America (2016-2018). Professor of Psychoneurocutaneous Medicine at the

University Deli Studi "G. Marconi" in Rome, Italy. She is a Faculty Member of the Institute for Bioethics and Health Policy, University of Miami Miller School of Medicine and a Volunteer Faculty- Associate Professor at the Department of Dermatology and Cutaneous Surgery, University of Miami Miller School of Medicine and Volunteer Faculty-Assistant Professor at the Department of Psychiatry and Behavioral Sciences, University of Miami Miller School of Medicine. Previously, she had a Research Fellowship in Dermatologic Surgery and Laser at the Department of Dermatology and Cutaneous Surgery, University of Miami Miller School of Medicine and a Fellowship in Cosmetic Medicine at the Department of Otorhinolaryngology and Facial Plastic Surgery, University of Miami Miller School of Medicine. She has over 100 scientific publications. She is the author of the textbook "Dermatology and Doctor-Patient Relationship" (Brazil, 2012), co- editor and author of "Geriatric Psychodermatology: Psychocutaneous Disorders in the Elderly" (USA, 2015) and co-author of "Optimal Patient Management of Alopecia" (United Kingdom, 2016). She has been invited as a speaker at major international conferences, including the European Academy of Dermatology Meeting, Congress of the Ibero-Latin American College of Dermatology, Kuwait Derma Update and Pediatric Dermatology Symposium, Brazilian Congress of Dermatology, among others. Her areas of expertise are Trichopsychodermatology, Geriatric Psychodermatology, Psychodermato-Oncology and Cosmetic Psychodermatology.

# MOHAMMAD JAFFERANY, MD

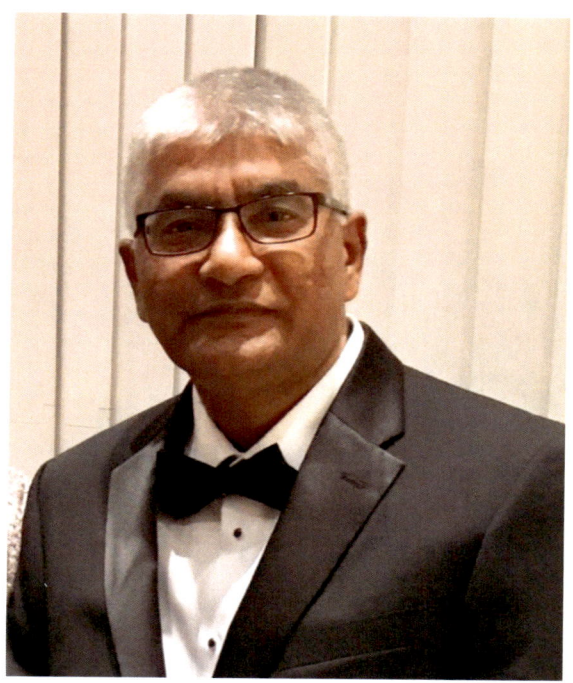

Dr. Mohammad Jafferany is a board certified Psychiatrist with dermatology training, who practices in Saginaw, Michigan. He is Clinical Associate Professor at Central Michigan University. He is Director Psychodermatology clinic at Jafferany Psychiatric Services and JPS Psychological Services. He did his adult Psychiatry residency at Hennepin County Medical Center in Minneapolis, Minnesota and fellowship in Child and Adolescent Psychiatry at University of Washington in Seattle, WA. Skin picking, trichotillomania and other psychocutaneous disorders are his particular interest. He is also Executive Secretary of Association for Psychocutaneous Medicine of North America, the national association for these disorders. He has numerous publications to his credit on various psychodermatological topics. He is the co-editor of books on Pediatric Psychodermatology, Geriatric Psychodermatology, Stress and Skin disorders and has written chapters on Psychocutaneous disorders in many books. He is a researcher, writer, lecturer and speaker in national and international conferences on psychodermatology.

# LIST OF CONTRIBUTORS

**José C. Cardoso, MD**
*Dermatology Department,*
Coimbra Hospital and University Centre
Coimbra, Portugal

**David Ernesto Castillo, MD**
*Department of Dermatology and Cutaneous Surgery*
University of Miami Miller School of Medicine
Miami, FL USA

**Enos Clinton, MD**
*Department of Internal medicine*
Eastern Virginia Medical School
Norfolk, VA, USA.

**Erin E. Curley, BA**
*Department of Psychiatry*
Massachusetts General Hospital/Harvard Medical School
Boston, MA, USA

**Bárbara R. Ferreira, MD**
*Dermatology Department,*
Coimbra Hospital and University Centre
Coimbra, Portugal

**Katlein França, MD, PhD**
*Centro Studi per la Ricerca Multidisciplinare e Rigenerativa*
Università Degli Studi "G. Marconi"
Rome, Italy

*Institute for Bioethics and Health Policy*
*Department of Dermatology and Cutaneous Surgery*
*Department of Psychiatry and Behavioral Sciences*
University of Miami Miller School of Medicine
Miami, FL USA

**Mohammad Jafferany, MD, FAPA**
*Department of Psychiatry*
Central Michigan University College of Medicine
Saginaw, MI, USA

*Jafferany Psychiatric Services and JPS Psychological Services*
Saginaw, MI, USA

**Nancy J. Keuthen, PhD**
*Department of Psychiatry*
Massachusetts General Hospital/Harvard Medical School,
Boston, MA, USA

**Angela Y. Kim, BS**
Nova Southeastern University College of Osteopathic Medicine,
Fort Lauderdale, FL, USA

**Torello Lotti, MD**
*Centro Studi per la Ricerca Multidisciplinare e Rigenerativa*
Università Degli Studi "G. Marconi"
Rome, Italy

**Ferdnand C. Osuagwu, MD**
*Department of Psychiatry*
Central Michigan University College of Medicine
Saginaw, Mi, USA

**José P. Reis, MD**
*Dermatology Department,*
Coimbra Hospital and University Centre
Coimbra, Portugal

**Jerry Shapiro, MD**
*The Robert O. Perelman Department of Dermatology*
New York University School of Medicine
New York, NY, USA

**Philip D. Shenefelt, MD**
*Department of Dermatology and Cutaneous Surgery*
University of South Florida
College of Medicine
Tampa, FL, USA

In: Trichotillomania (Hair Pulling Disorder)
Editors: K. França and M. Jafferany

ISBN: 978-1-53610-854-5
© 2017 Nova Science Publishers, Inc.

*Chapter 1*

# THE HISTORY OF TRICHOTILLOMANIA: THE BIBLE, SHAKESPEARE, AND OTHER CURIOSITIES

*Katlein França[1,2], MD, PhD, Angela Y. Kim[3], BS and Torello Lotti, MD[1]*

[1]Centro Studi per la Ricerca Multidisciplinare e Rigenerativa,
Universitá Degli Studi "G. Marconi," Rome, Italy
[2]Institute for Bioethics and Health Policy,
Department of Dermatology and Cutaneous Surgery,
Department of Psychiatry and Behavioral Sciences,
University of Miami Miller School of Medicine, Miami, FL, US
[3]Nova Southeastern University College of Osteopathic Medicine,
Fort Lauderdale, FL, US

## ABSTRACT

Trichotillomania (Hair Pulling Disorder) is an obsessive compulsive disorder characterized by an irresistible urge to pull out one's own hair leading to noticeable hair loss, distress, and social impairment according to the DSM-V criteria (Chattopadhyay 2012; Woods et al. 2014). As it is chronic and difficult to treat, trichotillomania is a challenging disorder for dermatologists (Enos and Plante 2001).

**Keywords**: trichotillomania, hair pulling disorder, history, trichopsychodermatology, psychodermatology

## SOCIALLY ACCEPTED RITUALS

The long history of trichotillomania is interesting and mysterious, with its story deeply rooted in various cultures, works of literature, art, and medicine. The act of intentional hair shaving, plucking, or pulling has long been described to be a ritual or a part of, certain societies (Stein et al. 1999). In ancient Greek, long locks of hair in men represented manliness and beauty. When there was a death of a friend or a relative, the Grecians would symbolize their physical presence surrounding the dead by piling some of their precious hair on top of their beloved corpse in funerals (Gillies 1786, 324). If long locks of hair signified attractive qualities of a man in Grecian culture, the act of sacrificing the hair to mound unto their dead family member or friend infers putting aside one's pride and paying respect to the dead.

Originated from India is a religion called Jainism, in which members must pull out their own hair as an initiation to become a monk or a nun in the sect. Jainism promotes renunciation of worldly desires and possessions. Ripping out one's own hair in a calm manner signifies the final transformation, determination and commitment in the religion (Whitney Kelting 2013, 86). In Jainism, hair plays a medium, through which the monks and nuns can express their willpower and pledge into the religion by enduring the painful plucking of all the hair from one's head.

In some Middle Eastern countries, brides are to remove all body hairs except for the hair on the head and eyebrows the night before the wedding as a custom. Similarly, there is a common practice of shaving and plucking body hair including pubic hair as a marriage ritual for some tribes in central Africa (Sherrow 2006, 180). Intentional hair removal in preparation for sacred ceremonies, such as matrimonies, may perhaps embody the concept of purity and innocence of a virgin. Moreover, removal of hair has indicated beauty for thousands of years. For example, the tombs of ancient Egypt contained cosmetic boxes with tweezers, which were used to pluck unwanted hair (Malam and Manning 2003, 28). As discussed above, these hair pulling and plucking rituals have been socially accepted as part of various cultures. However, trichotillomania has its own hairy history (Kim 2014).

## HAIR PULLING AS A SYMBOL OF GRIEF, FRUSTRATION, OR INSANITY

Aside from records of culturally accepted intentional hair pulling, implication of the relationship between hair pulling and grief, frustration, or insanity have been evident in many literary works for thousands of years. As the father of medicine and one of the earliest physicians recorded to date, Hippocrates has written seven books describing his observations and encounters with his patients. Written in the first book, *Epidemics 1*, is Hippocrates' advisory in including assessment of a patient for any hair pulling as part of a general health examination (Stein et al. 1999; Kim 2014):

> Then we must consider his speech, his mannerism, his silences, his thoughts, his habits of sleep or wakefulness and his dreams, their nature and time. Next, we must note whether he plucks his hair, scratches or weeps (Lloyd 1983, 100, quoted in Stein et al. 1999).

In grouping hair plucking, scratching and weeping together in the assessment, Hippocrates implies that the act of hair pulling is associated with confusion or sadness. In *Epidemics III*, Hippocrates describes a woman patient pulling out her hair in sorrow and depression (Stein et al. 1999; Kim 2014):

> At Thasos the wife of Delearces, who lay on the level ground, took a high fever with shivering as the result of grief. From the start she used to wrap herself up, always remaining silent while she groped about, scratching and plucking out hair and alternately wept and laughed (Lloyd 1983, p 137 quoted in Stein et al. 1999).

Other literary descriptions of trichotillomania can be found in the Bible, in works of William Shakespeare (Franca et al. 2013) and of Homer's The Iliad (Homer 1997). The book of Ezra in the bible indicates that marrying outside of the Hebrew community is considered an act of unfaithfulness to God. Upon finding out that many members of the Hebrew community, including priests, have been taking foreign wives, Ezra, a devout man of God, is frustrated, ashamed, and pulls out his hair. "At this news I tore my garment and my cloak; I tore hair from my head and beard and sat down, quite overcome (Ezra 9:3)." Ezra's anger toward the unfaithful Israelites and humility before God are portrayed through his act of tearing out his beard and hair from his head.

In Shakespeare's *Romeo and Juliet*, Romeo's world is shattered as Friar Laurence tells him he is banished for killing Tybalt, Juliet's cousin. Although Friar Laurence is trying to pacify Romeo that Prince's order of Romeo's banishment is better than death, Romeo continues to be in despair because he would not be able to see Juliet, whom he loves and just married an hour ago. Romeo argues that if Friar Laurence were to be Romeo banished away from Juliet, he too, would pull his hair out in sorrow:

> Thou canst not speak of that thou dost not feel. Wert thou as young as I, Juliet thy love. An hour but married, Tybalt murdered. Doting like me, and like me banished. Then mightst thou speak, then mightst thou tear thy hair. And fall upon the ground, as I do now. Taking the measure of an unmade grave (Romeo and Juliet, Act 3 Scene 3, quoted in Hylton, 1993).

The reference to tearing out the hair portrays Romeo's frustration and despair due to the thought of being physically separated from his love, Juliet. King John is another one of Shakespeare's works referencing hair pulling. A character named Constance pulls out her hair grieving for her son, who had been taken prisoner:

> I am not mad: this hair I tear is mine... Young Arthur is my son, and he is lost...I tore them from their bonds and cried aloud 'O that these hands would redeem my son, as they have given these hairs their liberty!' (King John, Act 3 Scene 4, quoted in Hylton 1993).

Constance states she is not crazy and that she pulls out her hair to show grief over her son. Like Ezra in the Bible, Constance's intentional act of tearing out hair seems to signify the desire to express her sincerity in the emotions she is overcome with. Rather than an act one wants done unto oneself, tearing out the hair becomes a symbolic display of distress. In *The Illiad*, Homer describes Agememnon, the King of Mycenae and commander-in-chief of his army against Troy, unable to sleep and in distress, which prompts him to pull out his hair:

> ... but Agamemnon son of Atreus was troubled...When he looked upon the plain of Troy he marveled at the many watchfires burning in front of Illius, and at the sound of pipes and flutes and of the hum of men, but when presently he turned towards the ships and hosts of the

Achaeans, he tore his hair by handfuls before Jove on high, and groaned aloud for the very disquietness of his soul (The Illiad, "Book X").

Other than in literary references, accounts of hair pulling are also portrayed in art works associated with emotional chaos. From the 8th century Grecian time are vase paintings of mourning women tearing out their hair (Kleiner 2013, 55). Similarly, in a painting in the Sienese Church of San Clemente ai Servi by Pietro Lorenzette in the 14th century of Italy, women are seen grieving by ripping out their hair and traumatizing their cheeks with their bare hands (Jacobus 1997, 47). Other works of art related to hair pulling imply overtone of insanity. Artist Artus Quellinus de Oude's The Women from the Mad House is a sculpture of a women pulling out her hair (Stein et al.1999). Another depiction of a mentally ill woman pulling her hair out in St. Luke's Asylum in London in 1809 is drawn by Thomas Rowlandson and August Pugin (Stein et al. 1999).

## EVOLUTION OF TRICHOTILLOMANIA AS A DISORDER IN DSM

Although described and spoken about for centuries, trichotillomania was not formally recognized as a mental disorder until it was included in Diagnostic and Statistical Manual of Mental Disorders (DSM)-III-Revised(R) in 1987 under the category of Impulse Control Disorder, Not Classified Elsewhere (APA, 1987). When DSM-III-R was updated to DSM-IV, trichotillomania remained categorized under Impulse Control Disorder Not Elsewhere Classified, together with pathological gambling, pyromania, intermittent explosive disorder, and kleptomania (APA, 1994). The major changes from DSM-III-R to DSM-IV included the addition of Criterion B: increased urge to pull out hair when trying to resist hair pulling and Criterion E: clinically significant distress or impairment in social, occupational, and other important areas of human functioning (Table 1).

A review article by Stein et al. (2010) suggested recommendations for changes in the classification of and criteria for trichotillomania for DSM-V. Among the recommendations was the reclassification of trichotillomania out of the Impulse Control Disorder Not Elsewhere Classified category, arguing that not all patients fit criteria B and C of DSM-IV. Not all patients felt the increase tension to pull out their hair nor felt relief, gratification, or pleasure out of the act (Stein et al. 2010). Furthermore, there were more differences than overlaps between other impulse control disorders, such as pathological gambling and intermittent explosive disorder, and trichotillomania. The review article proposed trichotillomania be classified as an obsessive compulsive spectrum disorder due to having more similarities in symptoms, comorbidities, and familial patterns with obsessive compulsive disorders than with impulsive control disorders. Ultimately, the new DSM-V published in 2013 reclassified trichotillomania under a new category of Obsessive-Compulsive and Related Disorders, along with hoarding disorder, excoriation (skin-picking) disorder, and body dysmorphic disorder (APA 2013a and APA 2013b).

With the reclassification of trichotillomania in DSM-V, criteria for hair pulling disorder have also been revised as criteria B and C in DSM-IV have been eliminated for the reasons mentioned previously. However, DSM-V still contain five criteria for hair pulling disorder (Table 2). In DSM-V, criterion B describes repeated attempts at hair pulling without the implication of increased urge to do the act. Moreover, criterion D in DSM-IV seems to be split into two criteria in DSM-V. Criterion D in DSM-V states that hair pulling but not be secondary to another medical condition and Criterion E, from another mental disorder.

**Table 1. DSM-IV diagnostic criteria for trichotillomania**

| |
|---|
| A. Recurrent pulling out one's hair resulting in noticeable hair loss |
| B. An increasing sense of tension immediately before pulling out the hair or when attempting to resist the behavior |
| C. Pleasure, gratification, or relief when pulling out the hair |
| D. The disturbance is not better accounted for by another mental disorder and is E. Not due to a general medical condition (e.g., a dermatological condition) |
| The disturbance causes clinically significant distress or impairment in social, occupational, or other important areas of functioning. |

**Table 2. DSM-V diagnostic criteria for trichotillomania**

| |
|---|
| A. Recurrent pulling out one's hair, resulting in hair loss |
| B. Repeated attempts to decrease or stop hair pulling |
| C. The hair pulling cause clinically significant distress or impairment in social, occupational, or other important areas of functioning. |
| D. The hair pulling or hair loss is not attributable to another medical condition (e.g., a dermatological condition). |
| E. The hair pulling is not better explained by symptoms of another mental disorder (e.g., attempts to improve a perceived defect or flaw in appearance in body dysmorphic disorder). |

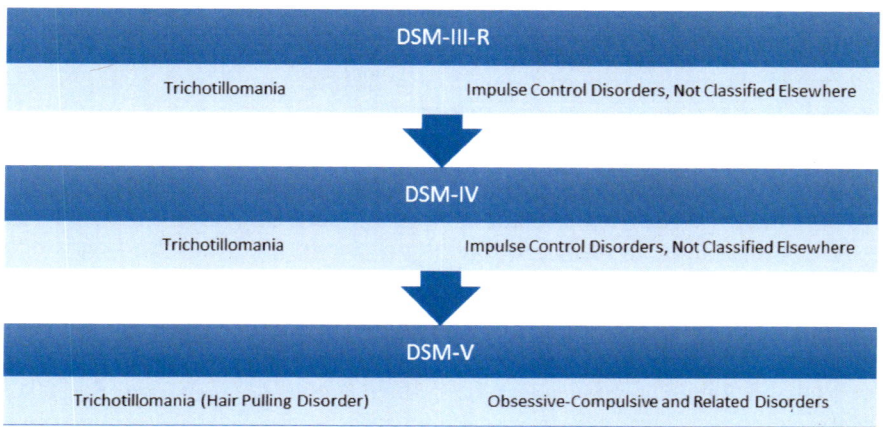

Figure 1. Evolution of Naming and Classification of Trichotillomania in the Diagnostic and Statistical Manual of Mental Disorders: DSM-V has reclassified trichotillomania under Obsessive-Compulsive and Related Disorder and now includes the sub-label of Hair Pulling Disorder.

Another recommendation made by Stein et al. (2010) was renaming trichotillomania as hair pulling disorder. The rationale behind this was that the word mania may further stigmatize the patient exacerbate the disorder by associating with other conditions, such as bipolar disorder. Subsequently, "Trichotillomania" in DSM-IV was renamed as "Trichotillomania (Hair Pulling Disorder)" with the sub label in parentheses in DSM-V (APA 2013b). Keeping the word trichotillomania in DSM-V was suggested to retain clinical and research continuity (Stein et al. 2010).

The evolution of trichotillomania, or hair pulling disorder, from DSM-III-R to DSM-V reveals the society's continuous effort to understanding the etiology and biology of the disorder (Figure 1). With records from ancient times, trichotillomania continues to divulge its mysterious origins. Hair pulling from emotional stress as depicted in literature, culture, art, and medicine is perhaps the key to understanding the current disorder, finding the root of its cause, and effectively managing those suffering from the disorder.

# REFERENCES

American Psychiatric Association (APA). Highlights of Changes from DSM-IV-TR to DSM-5. Arlington, VA: APA publishing, 2013a.

American Psychiatric Association (APA). "Obsessive-Compulsive and Related Disorders." Diagnostic and Statistical Manual of Mental Disoders. 5th ed. Arlington, VA: APA publishing, 2013b.

Chamberlain SR, Menzies L, Sahakian BJ, Fineberg NA. "Lifting the veil on trichotillomania." *Am J Psychiatry* 164, no. 4 (2007): 568–74. doi:10.1176/appi.ajp.164.4.568.

Chattopadhyay KI. "The genetic factors influencing the development of trichotillomania." *J Genet.* 91, no. 2 (2012): 259-62.

English Oxford Living Dictionaries. Oxford University Press, 2016. https://en.oxforddictionaries.com. Accessed November 26, 2016.

Enos SI, Plante T. "Trichotillomania: An overview and guide to understanding." *J Psychosoc Nurs Ment Health Serv.* 39, no. 5 (2001): 10-8.

França K, Chacon A, Ledon J, Savas J, Nouri K. "Psychodermatology: a trip through history." *Anais Brasileiros de Dermatologia.* 88, no. 5 (2013): 842-843. doi:10.1590/abd1806-4841.20132059.

Gillies J. "Chapter 7. History of Greece." The History of Ancient Greece, Its Colonies, and Conquests. Pg 324. London: Basil, 1786.

Homer. "Book X." The Iliad. Pg 121. Clayton, DE: Prestwick House, Inc, 1997.

Jacobus L. "Chapter 1 Motherhood and Massacre: The Massacre of the Innocents in Late-Medieval Art and Drama." The Massacre in History. Edited by Levene M and Roberts P. Pg 47. New York: Berghahn Books, 1999.

Kim WB. "On Trichotillomania and Its Hairy History." *JAMA Dermatol.* 150, no. 11 (2014): 1179. doi:10.1001/jamadermatol. 2014. 2284.

Kleiner FS. Gardner's Art Through the Ages: A Concise Global History. Pg55. Wadsworth, Cengage Learning, 2013

Malam J and Manning R. "Cosmetics and Beauty." Ancient Egyptian Women. Illustrated Ed. Pg 28. Chicago, IL: Reed Educational and Professional Publishing, 2003.

Shakespeare W. "The same. King Phillip's Tent." King John. Act 3 Scene 4. Quoted in Hylton J. The Life and Death of King John. The Complete Works of William Shakespeare. The Tech of MIT, 1993. http://shakespeare.mit.edu/john/john.3.4.html. Accessed November 26, 2016.

Shakespeare W. "Friar Laurence's cell." Romeo and Juliet. Act 3 Scene 3. Quoted in Hylton J. Romeo and Juliet. The Complete Works of William

Shakespeare. *The Tech of MIT*, 1993. http://shakespeare.mit.edu/romeo_juliet/romeo_juliet.3.3.html. Accessed November 26, 2016.

Sherrow V. "Hair Removal." Encyclopedia of Hair: A Cultural History. Pg 180. Westport, CT: Greenwood Press, 2006.

Stein DJ, Christenson GA, and Hollander E. Trichotillomania. Washington, DC: American Psychiatric Press, Inc, 1999.

Stein DJ, Grant JE, Franklin ME, Keuthen N, Lochner C, Singer HS, and Woods DW. "Trichotillomania (hair pulling disorder), skin picking disorder, and stereotypic movement." *Depression and Anxiety* 27 (2010): 611-626. doi: 10.1002/da.20700.

Whitney Kelting M. "Chapter 3: Jain traditions: Practicing tradition today." South Asian Religions: Tradition and Today. Edited by *Karen Pechilis and Selva J. Raj*. Pg 86. New York: Routledge, 2013.

Woods DW, Houghton DC. "Diagnosis, Evaluation, and Management of Trichotillomania." *The Psychiatric clinics of North America* 37, no. 3 (2014): 301-317. doi:10.1016/j.psc.2014.05.005.

In: Trichotillomania (Hair Pulling Disorder)  ISBN: 978-1-53610-854-5
Editors: K. França and M. Jafferany  © 2017 Nova Science Publishers, Inc.

*Chapter 2*

# TRICHOTILLOMANIA IN TRICHOPSYCHODERMATOLOGY

## *Katlein França*[\*], *MD, PhD*

Centro Studi per la Ricerca Multidisciplinare e Rigenerativa, Università Degli Studi "G. Marconi," Rome, Italy
Institute for Bioethics and Health Policy, Department of Dermatology and Cutaneous Surgery, Department of Psychiatry and Behavioral Sciences, University of Miami Miller School of Medicine, Miami, FL, US

### ABSTRACT

The emotional aspects of living with any hair disorder can be challenging [1]. Hair plays a multiplicity of roles. It is a means of projecting the image an individual has of him of herself. It is an object of traditions, culture, beliefs and behaviors and possesses powerful symbolic and evocative properties [2]. The hair shapes a person's identity. So it not surprising that any hair disorder that causes hair loss or excess of hair causes distress. Patients with hair disorders frequently present high levels of anxiety and depression [3]. Hair loss is a stressful experience for both sexes, but substantially more distressing for women. Women tend to place greater attention than men on physical appearance and attractiveness. The society suggests that hair fundamental part of a woman's sexuality as well as her gender identity [4]. A study performed with patients with hair loss in general practice found that 50% of patients

---

[\*] Corresponding author: E-mail: k.franca@med.miami.edu

had psychological problems. Male patients presented predominantly low self-esteem while female patients suffered predominantly of fear and anxiety [5]. Women are more likely than men to have a lowered quality of life and restrict social contacts due to hair loss [4, 6]. Excess of hair also can be a challenge for many. Diseases like hirsutism and hypetrichosis carries a high psychological burden and represents a significant intrusion into patient's daily lives [7].

The effect of stress on hair loss has been investigated by researchers and evidence suggests that neurohormones, neurotransmitters, and cytokines released during the stress response may influence the hair cycle [8]. Psychoemotional stress induces alteration of hair cycle through neuropeptide substance P (SP) mediated immune response. In a study performed in mice, the researchers demonstrated that chronic restraint stress alters the hair cycle by inhibiting hair follicle growth in vivo, prolonging the telogen stage and delaying subsequent anagen and catagen stage [9].

Once the patient develops the hair disorder he can develop psychological disturbances and a cycle, whereby psychological disturbances cause hair disorder and hair disorders cause psychological disorders, is created [10].

**Keywords**: trichopsychodermatology, trichotillomania, psychosocial impact, psychology, quality of life, psychotherapy

## INTRODUCTION

To address the different aspects of the psychosocial impact of hair disorders, the field called "Trichopsychodermatology" was created. Trichopsychodermatology is a subspecialty of psychodermatology. It is an emerging field of study, and studies the psychological and social impact of hair disorders, the effects of stress on hair loss, implementation of strategies to fight stigmatization and discrimination, depression and anxiety, improvement of the quality of life and the development of coping strategies and psychotherapy methods to patients affected by different hair disorders [1].

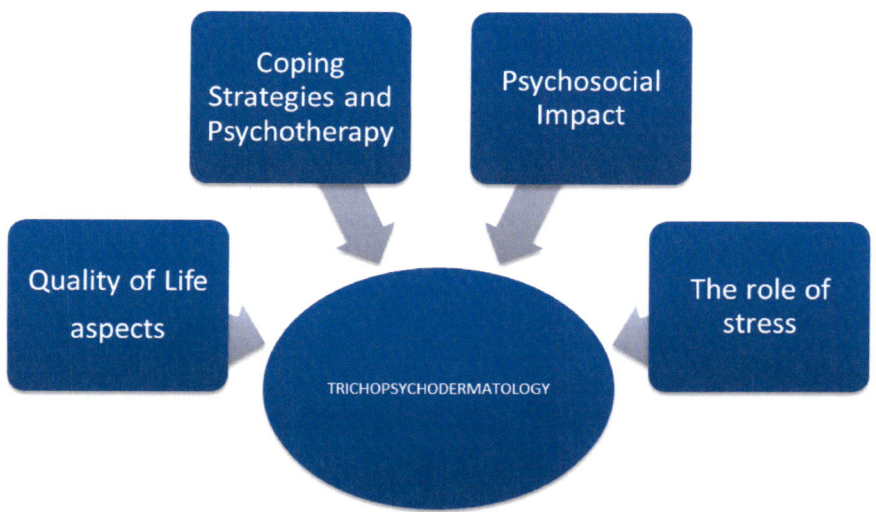

Scheme 1. Trichopsychodermatology and its areas of study.

## TRICHOTILLOMANIA IN THE CONTEXT OF TRICHOPSYCHODERMATOLOGY

Trichotillomania is one of the main diseases studied in the field of Trichopsychodermatology. Interactions between biological, environmental and psychological factors are important in development of hair pulling disorder [11].

This disease causes tremendous impact on patient's mental health and quality of life, particularly if it is left untreated [12]. Houghton et al. performed a study with 85 trichotillomania patients and found that 38.8% had another current psychiatric diagnosis and 78.8% had another lifetime (present and/or past) psychiatric diagnosis. Trichotillomania had substantial overlap with depressive, anxiety, addictive, and other body-focused repetitive behavior disorders. The authors also found that current depressive symptoms were the only predictor of quality of life deficits [13].

Trauma may play a role in development of trichotillomania but the duration of the disease seems to be correlated with decreased presence of post-traumatic stress symptoms. An interesting study performed by Özten et al. found that the reason for the negatively correlation of severity of post-traumatic stress symptoms and hair pulling disorder may be speculated as developing trichotillomania symptoms helps the patient to cope with intrusive thoughts related to trauma [11].

The relationship between violence and trichotillomania was investigated by Boughn et al. 91% of the sample studied by these authors reported some form or previous trauma or violence and 86% reported a history of violence concurrent with the onset of TTM. The events reported were sexual assault, rape and gang rape. These authors also speculated the possible relationship between family chaos experienced during childhood and the onset of TTM [14].

## CONCLUSION

Trichopsychodermatology is a subspecialty of psychodermatology and an upcoming field of study that is attracting attention from dermatologists and psychodermatologists worldwide. Hair loss is a stressful experience that can be stigmatizing for some patients and cause a severe psychological burden. Patients with hair disorders frequently present high levels of anxiety and depression. Trichotillomania is one of the main diseases studied in the field of Trichopsychodermatology. Psychiatric comorbidities are common among patients with Trichotillomania. This disease also has substantial overlap with depressive, anxiety, addictive, and other body-focused repetitive behavior disorders. Previous traumas and other situations involving violence may also play a role in the development of the disease. A detailed personal, familiar and medical history must be taken from each patient diagnosed with trichotillomania.

## REFERENCES

[1] França, K. et al. *Optimal Patient Management of Alopecia.* United Kingdom: GHC Communications (França, 2016).
[2] Sarode, B. and Beermann, F. (2009), Mysteries of salt and pepper. *Pigment Cell and Melanoma Research*, 22: 380-381.
[3] Hunt N, McHale S. The psychological impact of alopecia. *BMJ: British Medical Journal.* 2005;331(7522):951-953.

[4] Cash TF1, Price VH, Savin RC. Psychological effects of androgenetic alopecia on women: comparisons with balding men and with female control subjects. *J. Am. Acad. Dermatol.* 1993 Oct;29(4):568-75.

[5] de Koning EB1, Passchier J, Dekker FW. Psychological problems with hair loss in general practice and the treatment policies of general practitioners. *Psychol. Rep.* 1990 Dec;67(3 Pt 1):775-8.

[6] Van Neste DJ, Rushton DH. Hair problems in women. *Clin. Dermatol.* 1997;15:113-25.

[7] Lipton MG1, Sherr L, Elford J, Rustin MH, Clayton WJ. Women living with facial hair: the psychological and behavioral burden. *J. Psychosom. Res.* 2006 Aug;61(2):161-8.

[8] Paus R, Botchkarev VA, Botchkareva NV, Mecklenburg L, Luger T, Slominski A: The skin POMC system (SPS). Leads and lessons from the hair follicle. *Ann. NY Acad. Sci.* 1999, 885:350-363.

[9] Liu N1 et al. Chronic restraint stress inhibits hair growth via substance P mediated by reactive oxygen species in mice. *PLoS One.* 2013 Apr. 26;8 (4):e61574. doi: 10.1371/journal.pone.0061574. Print 2013.

[10] França K, Chacon A, Ledon J, Savas J, Nouri K. Pyschodermatology: a trip through history. *Anais Brasileiros de Dermatologia.* 2013;88(5): 842-843. doi:10.1590/abd1806-4841.20132059.

[11] Özten E, Sayar GH, Eryılmaz G, Kağan G, Işık S, Karamustafalıoğlu O. The relationship of psychological trauma with trichotillomania and skin picking. *Neuropsychiatric Disease and Treatment.* 2015;11:1203-1210. doi:10.2147/NDT.S79554.

[12] Diefenbach GJ1, Tolin DF, Hannan S, Crocetto J, Worhunsky P. Trichotillomania: impact on psychosocial functioning and quality of life. *Behav. Res. Ther.* 2005 Jul;43(7):869-84.

[13] Houghton DC1 Comorbidity and quality of life in adults with hair pulling disorder. *Psychiatry Res.* 2016 May 30;239:12-9. doi: 10.1016/j.psychres.2016.02.063. Epub. 2016 Mar. 2.

[14] Boughn S1, Holdom JJ. The relationship of violence and trichotillomania. *J. Nurs. Scholarsh.* 2003;35(2):165-70.

In: Trichotillomania (Hair Pulling Disorder)  ISBN: 978-1-53610-854-5
Editors: K. França and M. Jafferany  © 2017 Nova Science Publishers, Inc.

Chapter 3

# TRICHOTILLOMANIA: BASIC CONCEPTS

## Mohammad Jafferany[1,*], MD, FAPA and Ferdnand C. Osuagwu[2], MD

[1]Clinical Associate Professor of Psychiatry
Department of Psychiatry and Behavioral Sciences
College of Medicine, Central Michigan University, Saginaw, MI, US
[2]Department of Psychiatry and Behavioral Sciences, College of Medicine,
Central Michigan University, Saginaw, MI, US

### ABSTRACT

The word trichotillomania (hair pulling disorder) is derived from the Greek words *thrix* (hair), *tillein* (pulling out), and mania (madness). The term Trichotillomania was introduced in 1889 by French dermatologist Hallopeau. Trichotillomania was not officially included as a psychiatric disorder in DSM (diagnostic and statistical manual of mental disorder, by the American Psychiatric Association) until 1987, when it was classified as an impulsive control disorder, not elsewhere classified in the DSM III R. Currently in DSM V it is classified as an obsessive compulsive spectrum and related disorder. It is defined as recurrent pulling of one's own hair, leading to marked hair loss and functional impairment. (Table 1). Previous definitions of trichotillomania in DSM IV-TR included tension before pulling hair and a sense of relief and gratification after pulling out the hair, which have been dropped in current DSM V

---

[*] Corresponding author: Email: m.jafferany@cmich.edu

definition, based upon various studies. In a sample of 60 trichotillomania patients 17% did not report a mounting tension before pulling or tension release and pleasure or gratification associated with hair pulling [1]. In another study [2], when DSM criteria was strictly applied to a sample of 2579 college students, only 0.6% met the criteria of trichotillomania. When the criteria was broadened to include those who pulled hair but did not experience relief or gratification, the figure rose to 2.5%. Reeve and colleagues [3] found that only one subject experienced tension before hair pulling and relief after she completed pulling in a sample of 10 trichotillomania patients. Another study by King and colleagues [4] concluded that rising tension followed by relief or gratification may not be an appropriate diagnostic criterion.

## EPIDEMIOLOGY AND PREVALENCE

Very little systematized epidemiological research has been conducted so far. In a first systematic study of 2579 college freshman, Christenson et al. [2], found the lifetime prevalence of trichotillomania as 0.6%. Other studies noted point prevalence in the range of 0-3.9% [5, 6]. In another study, Rothbaum et al. [7] found that 11% of their sample reported chronic hair pulling, but only 1% reported chronically significant hair loss and distress. One epidemiological study form Israel interviewing 794 adolescents with trichotillomania, found the life time prevalence as 1% [8]. The mean age of trichotillomania is 13 years. The age of onset for hair pulling symptoms has been reported as bimodal, either in early childhood or in adolescence [9], It has been suggested that childhood onset of trichotillomania represents a relatively benign form, while late onset of Trichotillomania is more severe, resistant to treatment and associated with comorbid psychopathology [10, 11]. The female to male ratio is 4:1, however, in childhood the sex distribution appears to be equal [12]. This was also confirmed by Tay et al. [13] who conducted a retrospective study on 10 children. The mean age was 11.3 years and sex ratio was equal. Commonly affected site in their study was scalp. Associated findings were nail biting, skin picking, headaches, anxiety and nervousness. Golomb and Vavrichek [14] coined the Acronym "Fiddling Sheep" to explain the phenomenology and common findings noticed in children with trichotillomania. Fiddling sheep stands for "*F*iddling, *S*ensations, *H*ands, *E*motions, *E*nvironment, and *P*erfectionism. The family dynamic factors and onset triggers noted for trichotillomania include childhood illness and injury, death, illness or injury in the family, change in residence, alienation or separation from friends, entrance into school, academic difficulties, or school tension, onset of menarche, parental divorce, brief separation from parents, birth of siblings, sibling rivalry, poor marital relationship, and poor mother-child relationship.[15, 16, 17] Gershuny et al. [18] reported higher prevalence of Post-Traumatic Stress Disorder (PTSD) in trichotillomania than in the general population. 76% of their sample reported history of at least one traumatic event and 19% met the criteria of PTSD. The authors speculated that in traumatized individuals, trichotillomania may represent a form of coping or self-soothing strategy and the prevalence of PTSD in trichotillomania may be more than is expected on routine interview. Behavioral association with Trichotillomania has been noted as nail biting, cuticle biting, knuckle biting, thumb sucking, skin picking, picking at acne, nose picking, lip biting, cheek biting or chewing, face slapping, tongue chewing or biting, bruxism, face picking and clothes picking [19].

**Table 1. DSM-V Criteria of Trichotillomania**

| |
|---|
| A. Recurrent pulling out of one's own hair resulting in hair loss |
| B. Repeated attempts to decrease or stop hair pulling |
| C. The hair pulling causes clinically significant distress or impairment in social, occupational or other important areas of functioning |
| D. The hair pulling or hair loss is not contributable to another medical condition. (A dermatological condition). |
| E. The hair pulling is not better explained by its symptoms of another mental disorder (e.g., Attempts to improved perceived defect or flaw in appearance in Body Dysmorphic Disorder.) |

Two types of hair pulling have been described, known as automatic/habitual type, comprising of 5-47%, where hair pulling attention is focused elsewhere during the act of pulling. The other type is focused/compulsive type, and is comprised of 15-34%, where hair pulling attention is being expressly concentrated upon the act itself. Generally males with trichotillomania do not differ significantly from females, but males are twice likely to have obsessive compulsive spectrum Disorder. Association with body dysmorphic disorder, hypochondriasis, chronic motor tics, and Tourette syndrome have been reported frequently in males [20]. Trichotillomania could be familial as well. Swedo and Leonard [21] found 5% of first degree relatives had trichotillomania in a sample of 28 trichotillomania patients. Another study by Christenson et al. [22] reported 8% of first degree relative has trichotillomania in a sample of 161 patients. Post pulling manipulation of hair is common and includes stroking the hair against lips or face, biting of the root, examining the hair, playing with hair, chewing the hair and sometimes eating the hair [23]. The incidence of oral manipulation of hair has been reported in many patients with trichotillomania. Various studies have suggested the incidence from 5-77% and many hair pullers have different cues while pulling hair such as watching TV, reading, talking on the phone, lying in bed, drinking, writing, or doing paperwork [1]. Premenstrual exacerbations of urges to pull hair, which was alleviated during menstruations and thereafter was reported in a comprehensive study of 59 women [24]. Murphy et al. [25] suggested Trichotillomania as a form of NREM (non-rapid eye movement) sleep parasomnia, based upon a report of a 24year old women's video polysomnography showing rubbing of eyebrows in Stage 1 sleep and pulling eyelashes in Stage III and Stage IV sleep. A person with trichotillomania can pull hair at any body site with hair. (Figures 1 and 2). Woods et al. [26] found that scalp was the common site [72.8%] followed by eyelashes and eye brows [56.4%]. Other sites involved were pubic hair [50.7%], body hair and facial hair. The triggers to pull hair may be sensory, such as hair thickness, length and location and physical sensation on scalp. Emotional factors such as feeling anxious, bored, tense or angry also lead to pulling hairs. Cognitive factors including thoughts about hair and appearance, rigid thinking and cognitive errors also play a role in the production of hair pulling [27].

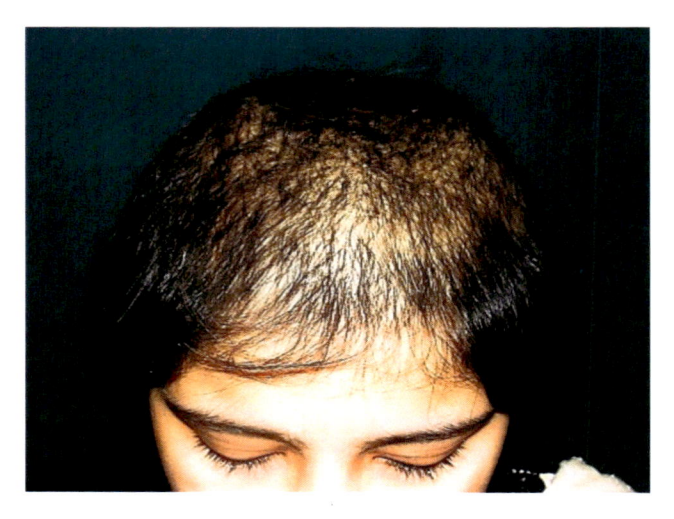

Figure 1. 18 years old girl with frontal Trichotillomania

# Trichotillomania: Basic Concepts 21

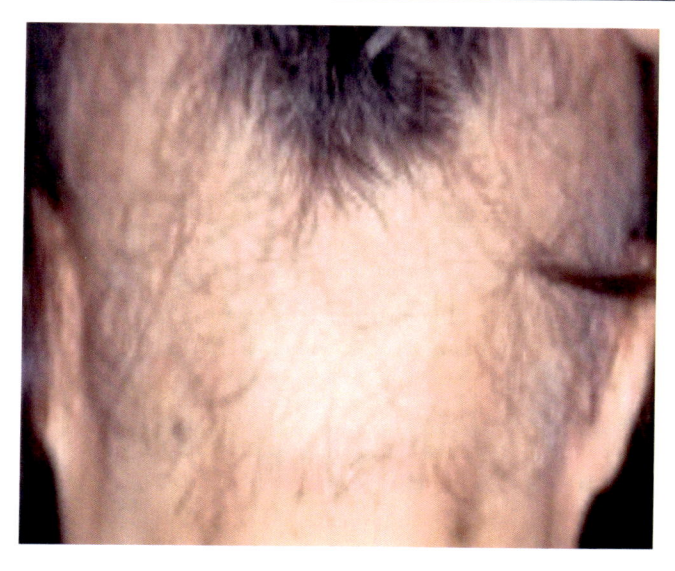

Figure 2. Significant hair loss on the back of scalp

A significant psychosocial dysfunction has been noted with patients with trichotillomania. Low self-esteem, depression, anxiety, guilt and shame is frequently associated with trichotillomania. In one study, almost one third of adults with trichotillomania reported low or very low quality of life [28]. Christenson et al. [29] reported that 87% of their patients attempted to disguise hair loss. Out of those 29% wore wigs, 36% wore scarves or hates and 51% styled their hair to cover the bald spots. Many patients avoid intimacy due to being "caught" by their partner, due to their bald patches. Many individuals avoid swimming for the same reason so that they could not be identified by people about their bald patches. Clinically patients with trichotillomania present with patches of hair loss or full alopecia. Pulling of hair in many patients may start in a wave like fashion across the scalp or centrifugally from a single standing point. Linear or circular patches with irregular boarders containing hair of varying length. Generally hair loss tends to occur on the contralateral side of the body from the dominant hand. The role of personality traits and their predictive validity for trichotillomania diagnosis, pulling severity and control and hair pulling style was investigated by Keuthen et al. [30]. The authors concluded that personality traits, especially neuroticism, can predict trichotillomania diagnosis, hair pulling severity and control and the focused style of pulling.

## DIFFERENTIAL DIAGNOSES

Many conditions mimic hair loss in trichotillomania. Obsessive compulsive disorder (OCD) is the most common differential diagnoses. Rates of OCD are significantly higher in individuals with trichotillomania. They range from 13-27% as reported in many studies [31, 32]. On the other hand, rates of trichotillomania among patients with OCD range from 5-7% [33, 34]. Although trichotillomania has been classified in Obsessive compulsive spectrum Disorder chapter in DSM –V, (Diagnostic and Statistical Manual of Mental Disorder by American Psychiatric Association) it has some common neurobiological pathways with OCD. Trichotillomania is a distinct form of OCD in many respects. Patients with trichotillomania are more likely to be females and they have higher rates of other body focused repetitive behavioral (BFRB) disorders such as skin picking or nail biting. These patients also have more first degree relatives with similar BFRB disorders. Compulsions in OCD are driven by intrusive thoughts, however, hair pulling is never driven by cognitive intrusions. Trichotillomania is commonly seen in early adolescence as compared to OCD which usually occurs in late adolescence. Both OCD and trichotillomania differ from the treatment point of view as well. Habit reversal therapy is the mainstay treatment for Trichotillomania, whereas exposure and response prevention are for OCD. SSRIs (selective serotonin reuptake inhibitors) are used for treatment for OCD, however SSRI may be used in trichotillomania but are not FDA recommended and efficacy is variable. Multiple forms of alopecia, different morphological hair disorders are also differentiated from trichotillomania on the clinical procedure. Anked et al. [35] used trichoscopy in 10 patients with trichotillomania. They found specific trichoscopic patterns including decreased hair density and broken hair and trichoptilosis (split ends) and irregular coiled hair in 80% patient. The authors conclude that trichoscopy plays a vital role in the diagnosis of trichotillomania by demonstrating specific trichoscopic patterns. Body dysmorphic disorder (BDD) sometimes counted in the differential diagnoses of trichotillomania. BDD is characterized by obsession and perceptions about a perceived defect of one's physical appearance. Hair pulling can occur in body dysmorphic disorder, but, its habit is motivated by the aim of correcting a perceived physical defect. Patients in BDD pull their hair on one side of the head to correct the perceived physical defect.

## COMORBIDITIES

Comorbidities in trichotillomania are norms rather than exception. A recent study by Flessnrer et al. [34] reported 60% of patients with trichotillomania may have some other psychiatric condition. A study conducted on children and adolescents showed that 64% of patients with Trichotillomania have at least one other diagnoses on Axis I [36]. The association between OCD and trichotillomania has been discussed in detail elsewhere in this chapter. Stewart et al. [37] reported 15.6% moderate hair pulling in OCD patients while 7.8% reported severe pulling with preponderance of the symptoms among women. Various studies have confirmed the association of trichotillomania with major depressive disorder, anxiety disorder and substance use disorder. Gunstad and Phillips [38] reported increased Axis I comorbidity correlation with more suicide attempts, lethality and more pronounced physical functional impairment. Woods et al. [26] did a landmark study of 894 patients with trichotillomania and found that 6% of patients had substance use problems. 17.7% patients used tobacco products and 14.1 used alcohol to relieve the negative feelings associated with hair pulling. The rate of anxiety was reported as 83% and depression due to hair pulling was reported as 70%. These high rates of anxiety and depression warrant physicians to screen every single patient with trichotillomania for psychiatric comorbidity and substance abuse. Miguel et al. [39] discussed the phenomenological differences in trichotillomania and Tourette's syndrome. The authors suggested that hair pulling and tics are repetitive behavior promoted by sensory cues and urges but not obsessions. O'Sullivan et al. [40] reported that morphometric MRI findings of Trichotillomania are similar to structural abnormalities associated with Tourette's syndrome.

## PATHOPHYSIOLOGY

Pathophysiology of Trichotillomania has been the subject of intense debate. No consensus on universally accepted cause been reached. Different etiological models have been proposed. Currently, trichotillomania has been classified under obsessive-compulsive spectrum disorder. Different hypothetical models suggested include psychoanalytical, biologic and behavioral models. Psychoanalytical models have been discussed in various studies. Tattersal [41] suggested trichotillomania as a symbolic expression of unconscious conflicts. Poor object relation theory was proposed by Krishnan et al. [42]. The authors suggest production of trichotillomania as a means of working through real or perceived threats of object loss. Singh and Maguire [43] focused on childhood trauma, physical and sexual abuse in cases of trichotillomania. The development of trichotillomania influenced by biologic and genetic factors remains unclear. Several authors reported 4-8% of first-degree relatives of trichotillomania patients as having hair pulling habits [1, 22]. Swedo and Leonard [21] have hypothesized the coexistence of a threshold for repetitive grooming behaviors, which could be lowered through the effects of stress or genetic susceptibility or triggered by autoimmune reaction.

Most of the research in the neurobiology of Trichotillomania has been centered on neuroanatomical studies looking for any brain abnormalities. Various studies have been conducted to find any structural abnormalities of the brain. Grachev [44] reported reduced left inferior frontal gyrus volumes and increased right cuneal volumes in patients with Trichotillomania as compared to healthy subjects. O'Sullivan et al. [40] reported similar left putamen volumes changes in trichotillomania patients as compared to healthy subjects Smaller cerebellar volumes in trichotillomania patients as compared to healthy individuals were also noted by Keuthen NJ et al. [45] Chamberlin and colleagues [46] reported higher gray matter density in several brain regions involved in affect regulation, motor habits, and cognition in individuals. Reduced thickness of right Para hippocampal gyrus in patients with trichotillomania, as compared to normal individuals was reported by Roos et al. [47]. Odlaug and associates [48] reported excess cortical thickness, not only in patient with trichotillomania but also in the in clinically asymptomatic first degree relatives, compared to healthy subjects with no known family history of Trichotillomania. White matter studies, using diffusion tensor imaging have shown lower fractional anisotropy in white matter tracts associated with the left and right anterior cingulate cortex, the left and right orbitofrontal cortex, the presupplementary motor area, the left primary somatosensory cortex and multiple temporal regions. These changes implicate disorganization of neurocircuitry involved in motor habit generation and suppression and effective regulation in patients with trichotillomania [49]. Functional neuroimaging studies have suggested dampening of nucleus accumbens responses to reward anticipation in patients with trichotillomania [50]. Lee et al. [51] did a pilot study of brain activation in children with trichotillomania during a visual-tactile symptom provocation task. The authors reported that patients with Trichotillomania demonstrated significantly greater activation in the left temporal cortex, the dorsal posterior cingulate gyrus and the putamen during visual symptom provocation and greater activation in the precuneus and dorsal posterior cingulate gyrus during visual and tactile provocation.

The genetic basis of Trichotillomania is still in infancy. Various genetic studies have shown associations with Trichotillomania. Synapse-associated protein 90/post-synaptic density protein 95-associated protein 3 (SAPAP3) is an excitatory postsynaptic protein seen in obsessive compulsive behaviors. Many studies have suggested that genetic deletion of SAPAP 3 causes OCD like behaviors [52]. Variants of SAPAP3 have been implicated in the etiology of OCD and Trichotillomania among South African adults [53]. Other genetic studies have suggested mutation and sequence variation in SLIT and TRK like 1. (SLITRK1) gene [54]. Abelson et al. [55] identified a frameshift mutation in micro RNA binding site variation in there independent Tourette's syndrome families. The mother of one proband carried the SLITRK1 mutation and was diagnoses with Trichotillomania. Another gene thought to having potential role in the etiology of Trichotillomania is the Hoxb8 gene. Studies conducted on mice have shown that Hoxb8 homozygous mutant mice were observed to demonstrate repetitive grooming behaviors on themselves and their cage-mates with excessive hair shedding [56].

Behavioral models of Trichotillomania includes tension reduction theory as suggested by Azrin and Nunn [57]. They proposed that hair pulling is thought to develop as a coping behavior in response to stress and is reinforced by means of tension reduction. Watson and Allen [58] discussed response covariation theory. They noted that thumb sucking and hair pulling have been observed to co-vary in children. They suggested successful treatment of thumb sucking has eliminated covariant hair pulling. This is more useful in early onset childhood trichotillomania. Modeling theory was postulated by Christenson et al. [22]. They suggested that hair pulling may be facilitated through observational learning process.

Different variants of trichotillomania have been described in literature. Trichorrizophagia, where patients eat the roots of plucked hair. Here patients have irresistible compulsion to pull out or twist and break off one's own hair. Extracted hair are often manipulated, examined or played with before being discarded or eaten [59]. Trichotemnomania is the compulsive habit to remove the hair of the scalp, eyebrows, axillary and pubic areas by compulsive shaving [60]. Trichoteiromania is the condition where patients compulsively rub on a part of the scalp to produce a bald patch. Constant rubbing results in fracturing of the hair. Light microscopy of the hair shafts show split brush like ends of otherwise normal hair [61]. Another recent condition described by

Jafferany et al. [62] and coined the term trichodaganomania. In this condition, the subjects compulsively bite their own hair on areas like forearm, and produce bald patches. Trichotillomania may also result in various medical complications. Pulling of hair can lead to skin damage if tweezers and scissors are used. Besides biting the roots of hair, many individuals with trichotillomania ingest their hair. This results in gastrointestinal hair balls called Trichobezoars, which may obstruct the gastrointestinal tract, leading to surgical intervention [63]. Patients with trichotillomania may also report blepharitis, chronic neck, back, or shoulder pain, and carpel tunnel syndrome due to abnormal pulling postures. Some patients avoid health care to escape shame and embarrassment.

## ASSESSMENT TOOLS/SCREENING/SCALES

Due to a specific behavioral pattern, trichotillomania is not difficult to diagnose. Trichotillomania is a chronic illness with fluctuations in intensity over time. Due to shame, guilt and embarrassment associated with trichotillomania, many patients try to avoid seeking treatment. In a study on 1048 patients who met the diagnostic criteria for Trichotillomania, only 39.5% had received treatment from a Therapist and only 27.3% had sought treatment from a psychiatrist [26]. Besides clinical interview, several measures and screening tools have been used in diagnosing and managing treatment response, finding comorbidities and self-monitoring. Table 2 shows various assessment tools and scales used.

Histopathological findings in Trichotillomania include empty antigen follicles, increased number of non-inflamed antigen follicles and pigment casts, mild perivascular lymphocytic infiltrate and incompletely keratinized distorted and pigmented hair shafts.

## Prognosis

Trichotillomania is characterized by exacerbation and remissions. In most cases this condition is chronic with fluctuations in intensity over time. The remitting and chronic form is related to age at onset and sex of the patient. Adolescent female patients are more susceptible to chronic form.

### Table 2. Assessment tools, Screening and Scales

| | |
|---|---|
| 1. | Diagnostic Modules: |
| | Trichotillomania diagnostic Interview |
| | Minnesota Trichotillomania Assessment Inventory-II (MTAI-II) |
| 2. | Clinician-rated Measures |
| | National Institute of Mental Health Trichotillomania severity scale (NIMH-TSS) |
| | National Institute of Mental Health Trichotillomania impairment scale (NIMH-TIS) |
| | Psychiatric Institute Trichotillomania Scale (PITS) |
| | Yale –Brown Obsessive Compulsive Scale-Trichotillomania (Y-BOCS-TTM) |
| 3. | Self-Report Measures |
| | Cues Check list |
| | Massachusetts General Hospital Hair pulling scale (MGH-HPS) |
| | Milwaukee Inventory for subtypes of trichotillomania- Adult version (MIST-A) |
| | Milwaukee Inventory for styles of trichotillomania- Child version (MIST-C) |
| | Trichotillomania Scale for Children (TSC) |
| | Milwaukee Dimensions of trichotillomania scale (M-DOTS) |
| 4. | Self-Monitoring |
| | Saving pulled hair |
| | Keeping daily records (self-monitoring forms) |
| 5. | Collateral Reports |
| | From family members |
| | For children and intellectually deficient patients |
| 6. | Objective Measures |
| | Pre and Post-treatment photographs |

## Treatment

Until now, there is no FDA approved medication for trichotillomania on the shelf. Behavioral therapy, mainly habit reversal therapy, combined with pharmacological treatment has shown positive outcome. Dougherty et al. [64] in a randomized double blind study suggested combination therapy with SSRI and habit reversal therapy may be more efficacious in the treatment of trichotillomania than either approach alone. In preschool year, trichotillomania is considered as a habit disorder, analogous to thumb sucking and expected to disappear by its own. Parental support and education about this benign course of disorder should be discussed with parents. In school age years, behavioral approaches have been found more efficacious that pharmacological therapy. In this age group, because of possibility of comorbid psychiatric disorder and psychiatric referral is warranted. In adolescent and adult, combination of pharmacotherapy, behavioral therapy and treatment of comorbid psychiatric disorders, if any, offers the most clinical benefit.

The behavioral treatment with the strongest empirical support is habit reversal therapy. However, other concomitant techniques including self-monitoring, coping strategies, motivation enhancement, stimulus control, relaxation training, token programs and use of transitional objects have also been used. Habit reversal therapy is considered the mainstay of treatment of trichotillomania. The major components of habit reversal therapy include self-monitoring and awareness training, competing response procedures and stimulus control. In awareness training, patient is given self-monitoring form, where she/he would document her/his location of pulling, preceding feelings and emotions, urges to pull and resist, number of times pulled and possible triggering or aggravating factors. The second component of habit reversal therapy is competing response training. Here patient is taught to compete the urge of pulling hair with another benign action. Patients then replace the pulling action into another act which is not harmful. The third component of habit reversal therapy is stimulus control procedures. Patients are educated to modify the environment to reduce cues for hair pulling. Within each of these components the patient learns to recognize his or her pulling urges, avoid situations in which pulling is more likely and adopt behaviors that can be used instead of pulling. Habit reversal therapy is simple, effective and easy to use. It can be delivered in person in a session of 45-60 minutes, online using a self-help method or in group format. Marcks et al. [65] conducted a postal survey on trichotillomania related knowledge and awareness in 501 general practitioners, psychiatrists and psychologists nationwide. Authors concluded that participants were fairly accurate about the effectiveness of treatment strategies, however an overwhelming majority of providers did not have any resources or referral information available for patients.

Although, there is no FDA approved pharmacological agent, SSRIs (Selective Serotonin Reuptake Inhibitors) are currently the most popular agents being used by many providers with variable success. Augmentation strategies with antipsychotics, anxiolytics, tricyclic antidepressants, lithium, naltrexone, topical steroids and topical capsaicin have been described in literature. A Cochrane database systemic review [66] reported no strong evidence of treatment benefit with SSRIs. Recently interest has grown in glutamatergic agents such as N-Acetylcysteine [NAC]. Grant et al. [67] in a double blind placebo controlled study demonstrated benefit in patients with trichotillomania at 1200 mg twice a day dose for nine weeks. Another randomized double blind placebo controlled study of Olanzapine [68] reported a significant reduction in symptoms of trichotillomania at a mean dose of 10.8 mg a day in 12-week period. Recently Dronabinol, a cannabinoid agonist has raised interest in the treatment of trichotillomania. In a pilot study Dronabinol was used with the mean dose of 11.6 mg per day during a 12-week trial period. Authors report marked reduction in symptoms of trichotillomania [69]. In a systematic review [70] on the treatment of trichotillomania, authors conclude that habit reversal therapy is the most effective intervention for trichotillomania. Clomipramine also showed benefit for symptoms of trichotillomania, while SSRIs did not appear to be effective.

The management of patients with trichotillomania require a comprehensive treatment plan involving patient and family and taking into consideration the whole picture [71]. The management guidelines conducting a thorough psychiatric examination and assessing for any comorbid psychiatric disorder such as depression, anxiety, mood disorder or obsessive compulsive disorder. Medical examination is also recommended particularly for possible trichobeazoars or hair ingestion or associated gastrointestinal symptoms, if history points to that. During first time evaluation patient and family should be educated about the nature of problem, possible etiologic factors, triggering factors, treatment options and risks and benefits associated with individual treatment options. (Figure 3). Patients and family should be informed about the newest research medications such as NAC, Dronabinol and also provided with community resources such as TLC foundation for body focused repetitive behavior disorders (www.trich.org). On this website patients and families could get educational material and can find the names and contact information of providers who are specialized in the treatment of trichotillomania by geographic preference.

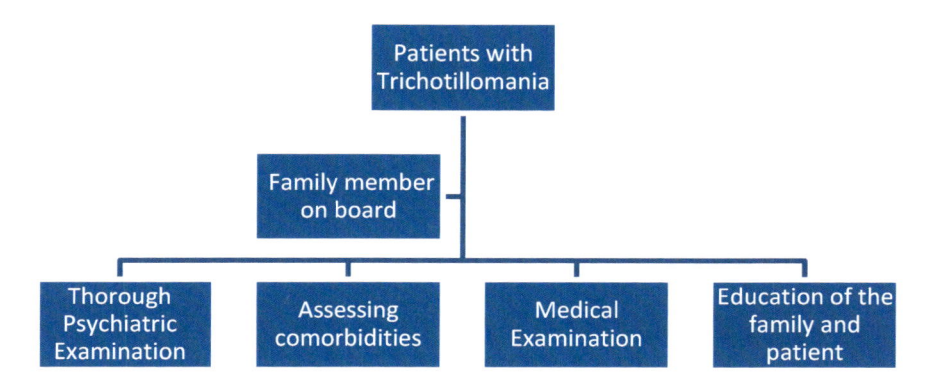

Figure 3. Management Guidelines.

## REFERENCES

[1] Christenson GA, Mackenzie TB and Mitchell JE. Characteristics of 60 adult chronic hair pullers. *Am J Psych.* 1991. 148:365-370.

[2] Christenson GA, Pyle RL and Mitchell JE. Estimated life time prevalence of trichotillomania in college students. *J Clin Psychaitry.* 1991.52:415-417.

[3] . Reeve EA, Bernstein GA and Christenson GA. Clinical characteristics and psychiatric comorbidity in children with trichotillomania. *J Am Acad Child Adolesc Psychiatry.* 1992. 31(1):132-381.

[4] King RA, Scahill L, Vitulano LA et al. Childhood trichotillomania: clinical phenomenology, comorbidity and family genetics. *J Am Acad Child Adolesc Psychiatry.* 1995. 34(11):1451-59.

[5] Odlaug BL, Grant JE. Impulse control disorders in a college sample: results from the self-administered Minnesota Impulse Disorders Interview (MIDI). *Or Care Companion J Clin Psychiatry* 2010; 12 (doi: 10.4088/PCC.09m00842whi).

[6] Manseuto CS, Thomas AM, Brice AL. Hair pulling and its affective correlates in an African-American University sample. *J Anxiety Disord* 2007; 21:590-99.

[7] Rothbaum BO, Shaw L, Morris R et al. Prevalence of trichotillomania in a college freshmen population.(Letter to Editor) *J Clin Psychiatry.* 1993. 54:72.

[8] King RA, Zohar AH, Ratzoni G et al. An epidemiological study of trichotillomania in Israeli adolescents. *J Am Acad Child Adolesc Psychiatry.* 1995; 34:1212-1215.

[9] Swedo SE and Rapoport JL. Annotation: Trichotillomania. *J Child Psychology Psychiatry.* 1991. 32:401-409.

[10] Swedo SE and Leonard HL. Trichotillomania: An obsessive compulsive spectrum disorder? *Psychiatr Clin North Am.* 1992. 15:777-790.

[11] Winchel RM. Trichotillomania: Presentation and treatment. *Psychiatric Annals.* 1992. 22:84-89.

[12] Lewin AB, Piacentini J, Flessner CA et al. Depression, anxiety and functional impairment in children with trichotillomania. *Depress Anxiety.* 2009; 26:521-27.

[13] Tay, YK, Levy, ML and Metry DW. Trichotillomania in children: Case series and review. *Pediatrics.* 2004; 113:494-4.

[14] Golomb, RG, Vavrichek SM. *The hair pulling habit and you: How to solve the trichotillomania puzzle.* Silver Springs, MD. Writers' cooperative of greater Washington. 2000.

[15] Muller SA. *Trichotillomania. Dermatol Clin.* 1987. 5:595-601.

[16] Slagle DA. Martin TA. Trichotillomania. *Am Fam Physician.* 1991. 43:2019-24.

[17] Adam BS, Kashani JH. Trichotillomania in children and adolescents: review of the literature and case report. *Child Psychiatry Hum Dev.* 1990. 20:159-63.

[18] Gershuny BS, Keuthen NJ, Gentes EL et al. Current post traumatic stress disorder and history of trauma in trichotillomania. *J Clinical Psychol.* 2006; 62(12):1521-29.

[19] Simeon D, Cohen LJ, Stein DJ. Comorbid self-injurious behaviors in 71 female hair pullers: a survey study. *J Nerv Ment Dis.* 1997. 185:117-9.

[20] Christenson GA, Mackenzie TB, Mitchell JE. Adult men and women with trichotillomania. A comparison of male and female characteristics. *Psychosomatics.* 1994; 35:142-49.

[21] Swedo SE and Leonard HL. Trichotillomania: an obsessive-compulsive spectrum disorder. *Psychiatr Clin North Am.* 1992; 15:777-790.

[22] Christenson GA, Mackenzie TB and Reeve EA. Familial trichotillomania. (Letter). *Am J Psychiatry.* 1992; 149:283.

[23] Schlosser S, Black DW, Blum N, Goldstein RB. The demography, phenomenology and family history of 22 persons with compulsive hair pulling. *Ann Clin Psychiatry.* 1994 6:147-52.

[24] Keuthen NJ, O'sullivan RL et al. The relationship of menstrual cycle and pregnancy to compulsive hairpulling. *Psychother Psychosom.* 1997. 66(1):33-37.

[25] Murphy C, Valerio T and Zallek SN. Trichotillomania: A NREM sleep parasomnia? *Neurology.* 2006; 66(8):1276.

[26] Woods DW, Flessner CA, Franklin ME et al. The trichotillomania impact project (TIP): exploring phenomenology, functional impairment and treatment utilization. *J Clin Psychiatry.* 2006; 67:1877-88.

[27] Christenson GA. Trichotillomania: from prevalence to comorbidity. *Psychiatr Times* 1995; 12:44-48.

[28] Odlaug BL, Kim SW, Grant JE. Quality of life and clinical severity in pathological skin picking and trichotillomania. *J Anxiety Disord.* 2010; 24:823-829.

[29] Christenson GA, Manseuto CS. *Trichotillomania: descriptive characteristics and phenomenology, in Trichotillomania.* Edited by

Stein DJ, Christianson GA, Hollander E. Washington DC, American Psychiatric Press, 1999, pp1-41.

[30] Keuthen NJ, Tung ES, Altenburger EM et al. Trichotillomania and personality traits from the five factor model. *Rev Bras Psiquiatr.* 2015; 37(4):317-24.

[31] Swedo SE, Leonard HL. Trichotillomania: an obsessive-compulsive spectrum disorder? *Psychiatr Clin North Am.* 1992; 15:777-790.

[32] Lovato L, Ferrao YA, Stein DJ et al. Skin picking and trichotillomania in adults with obsessive-compulsive disorder. *Compr Psychiatry.* 2012; 53:562-568.

[33] Torresan RC, Ramos-Cerqueria AT, Shavitt RG et al. Symptom dimensions, clinical course and comorbidity in men and women with obsessive-compulsive disorder. *Psychiatry Res.* 2013; 209:186-195.

[34] Flessner CA, Knopic VS, McGeary J. Hair pulling disorder (trichotillomania): genes, neurobiology and model for understanding impulsivity and compulsivity. *Psychiatry Res.* 2012; 199(3): 151-58.

[35] Anked BS, Naidu MV, Beergouder SL et al. Trichoscopy in trichotillomania: a useful diagnostic tool. *In J Trichology.* 2014; 6(4):160-63).

[36] Hana GL. Trichotillomania and related disorders in children and adolescents. *Child Psychiatry and Human Development.* 1997; 27(4): 255-268.

[37] Stewart SE, Jenike MA, Keuthen NJ. Severe obsessive compulsive disorder with and without comorbid hair pulling: comparisons and clinical implications. *J Clin Psychiatry.* 2005; 66(7):864-69.

[38] Gunstad J, Phillips KA. Axis I comorbidity in body dysmorphic disorder. *Compr Psychiatry.* 2003; 44:270-276.

[39] Miguel EC, Baer L, Coffey BJ et al. Phenomenological differences appearing with repetitive behavior in OCD and Tourette's syndrome. *Brit J Derm.* 1997; 170:140-45.

[40] O'Sullivan RL, Rauch SL, Breiter HC et al. Reduced basal ganglia volumes in trichotillomania measured via morphometric magnetic resonance imaging. *Biol Psychiatry.* 1997; 42:39-45.

[41] Tattersal ML. Further comments on trichotillomania (Letter to Editor) *Am J Psychiatry.* 1992. 149:284.

[42] Krishnan KRR, Davidson JRT, Guajardo C. Trichotillomania: A review. *Comp Psychiatry.* 1985. 26:123-28.

[43] Singh AN, Maguire J. Trichotillomania and incest. *Brit J Dermatol.* 1989; 155:108-10.

[44] Grachev ID. MRI-based morphometric topographic parcellation of human neocortex in trichotillomania. *Psychiatry Clin Neuroscience.* 1997; 51-315-321.
[45] Keuthen NJ, Makris N, Schlerf JE et al. Evidence for reduced cerebellar volumes in trichotillomania. *Biol Psychiatry.* 2007; 61:374-381.
[46] Chamberlain SR, Menzies LA, Fineberg LA et al. Grey matter abnormalities in trichotillomania: morphometric magnetic resonance imaging study. *Br J Psychiatry.* 2008; 193:216-221.
[47] Roos A, Grant JE, Fouche JP et al. A comparison of brain volume and cortical thickness in excoriation (skin picking) disorder and trichotillomania (hair pulling disorder) in women. *Behav Brain Res* 2015; 279:255-258.
[48] Odlaug BL, Chamberlain SR, Derbyshire KL et al. Impaired response inhibition and excess cortical thickness as candidate endophenotypes for trichotillomania. *J Psychiatr Res* 2014;59:167-173.
[49] Chamberlain SR, Hampshire A, Menzies LA et al. Reduced brain white matter integrity in trichotillomania: a diffusion tensor imaging study. Arch Gen Psychiatry 2010;67:965-971.
[50] White MP, Shirer WR, Molfino MJ et al. Disordered reward processing and functional connectivity in trichotillomania: a pilot study. *J Psychiatr Res* 2013; 47:1264-1272.
[51] Lee JA, Kim CK, Jahng GH et al. A pilot study of brain activation in children with trichotillomania during a visual-tactile symptom provocation task: a functional magnetic resonance imaging study. *Prog Neuropsychopharmacol Biol Psychiatry* 2010; 34:1250-1258.
[52] Wan Y, Ade KK, Caffall Z et al. Circuit selective striatal synaptic dysfunction in the SAPAP3 knockout mouse model of obsessive compulsive disorder. *Biol Psychiatry* 2014; 75(8): 623-30.
[53] Boardman L, Marwe LVD, Lochner C et al. Investigating SAPAP3 variants in the etiology of obsessive-compulsive disorder and trichotillomania in the South African White population. *Compr Psychiatry* 2011; 52(2):181-187.
[54] Zuchner S, Cuccaro ML, Tran-Viet KN et al. Slitrk1 mutations in trichotillomania. *Molecular Psychiatry.* 2006; 11(10):887-889.
[55] Abelson JF, Kwan KY, Roak BJO et al. Sequence variants in SLITRK1 are associated with Tourette's Syndrome. *Science* 2005; 310(5746):317-20.
[56] Greer JM and Capecchi MR. Hoxb8 is required for normal grooming behavior in mice. *Neuron.* 2002; 33(1):23-34.

[57] Azrin NH and Nunn RG. Habit reversal: A method of eliminating nervous habits and tics. *Behav Res Ther.* 1973; 11:619-628.
[58] Waston TS and Allen KD. Elimination of thumb sucking as a treatment for severe trichotillomania. *J Am Acad Child Adolesc Psychiatry* 1993; 32:830-34.
[59] Grimalt R, Happle R. Trichorrizophagia. *Eur J Dermatol* 2004; 14(4):266-7.
[60] Happle R. Trichotemnomania: obsessive compulsive habit of cutting or shaving the hair. *J Am Acad Dermatol* 2005; 52:157-59.
[61] Freyschmidt-Paul P, Hoffman R, Happle R. Trichoteiromania. *Eur J Dermatol* 2001; 11(4):369-71.
[62] Jafferany M, Feng J, Hornung R. Trichodaganomania; a compulsive habit of biting one's own hair. *J Am Acad Dermatol* 2009; 60(4):689-91.
[63] Grant JE, Odlaug BL. Clinical characteristics of trichotillomania with trichophagia. *Compr Psychiatry* 2008; 49:579-584.
[64] Dougherty DD, Loh R, Jenike MA et al. Single modality versus dual modality treatment for trichotillomania: Sertraline, behavioral therapy or both. *J Clin Psychiatry* 2006; 67(7):1086-92.
[65] Marcks BA, Wetterneck, CT and Woods DW. Investigating healthcare providers' knowledge of trichotillomania and its treatment. *Cogn Behav Ther* 2006; 35:19-27.
[66] Rothbart R, Amos T, Siegfried N et al. Pharmacotherapy for trichotillomania. *Cochrane database Sys Rev.* 2013; 11:CD007662.
[67] Grant JE, Odlaug BL, Kim SW. N-Acetylcysteine, a glutamate modulator in the treatment of trichotillomania: a double blind placebo controlled study. *Arch Gen Psychiatry* 2009; 66:756-763.
[68] Van Ameringen M, Mancini C, Patterson B et al. A randomized double blind placebo controlled trial of Olanzapine in the treatment of trichotillomania. *J Clin Psychiatry* 2010; 71:1336-1343.
[69] Grant JE, Odlaug BL, Chamberlain SR et al. Dronabinol, a cannabinoid agonist, reduces hair pulling in trichotillomania: a pilot study. *Psychopharmacology (Berl)* 2011;218:493-502.
[70] Bloch MH, Landros-Weisenberger A, Dombrowski P. et al. Systamatic review: pharmacological and behavioral treatment for trichotillomania. *Biol Psychiatry* 2007;62(8):839-46.
[71] Grant JE, Chamberlain SR. Trichotillomania. *AmJ Psychiatry* 2016; 173(9):868-74.

In: Trichotillomania (Hair Pulling Disorder)     ISBN: 978-1-53610-854-5
Editors: K. França and M. Jafferany     © 2017 Nova Science Publishers, Inc.

**Chapter 4**

# DERMATOPATHOLOGY AND TRICHOTILLOMANIA

## *Bárbara Roque Ferreira, MD, José Pedro Reis, MD and José Carlos Cardoso, MD*[*]

Dermatology Department, Coimbra Hospital and University Centre, Coimbra, Portugal

### ABSTRACT

Trichotillomania, resulting from self-induced pulling of hair, is a traumatic etiology of hair loss, in the group of traction and pressure alopecia. Histopathological findings are typically those of a non-scarring alopecia but, depending on the duration, it may develop some features of scarring alopecia, especially in cases of longstanding disease. Trichotillomania displays some distinctive histopathological features, which, although often subtle, may help to confirm the diagnosis in cases with difficult clinical presentation. The most characteristic findings are the distortion of hair follicles (trichomalacia) and the presence of pigment casts. This chapter presents the main clinical differential diagnoses of trichotillomania that may raise difficulties to ascertain the diagnosis and discusses how histopathology can be helpful. The types of alopecia that may share features with trichotillomania are also discussed, highlighting the similarities and differences that can be useful to establish the diagnosis of trichotillomania in challenging cases.

---

[*] Corresponding author: E-mail: jose.c.cardoso@gmail.com

## 1. INTRODUCTION

Trichotillomania is the most common pathological and compulsive skin-picking syndrome. Some authors have also suggested that some patients may also have impulsive features [1]. Although patients with trichotillomania commonly have a bizarre pattern of alopecia (one or more patches of incomplete alopecia, with irregular shape), in a few cases the clinical presentation may pose a considerable diagnostic challenge, raising other clinical differential diagnoses [2]. Globally considered, diseases of the hair are usually linked with high impact on body image and self-esteem, which should not be underestimated, particularly by clinicians. Therefore, their correct diagnosis is of utmost importance [3]. In this chapter, we will discuss the main clinical and histopathological alopecias (scarring and non-scarring), which belong to the differential diagnoses of trichotillomania. Firstly, we will present the main basic concepts behind this matter.

Alopecias are classified in "non-scarring" and "scarring" or "cicatricial," relating the term "scarring" to "permanent." Trichotillomania, alopecia areata, congenital triangular alopecia are examples of non-scarring type. In turn, classic pseudopelade and lichen planopilaris are examples of scarring types. Despite this classification, some non-scarring alopecias may also be permanent, such as alopecia areata, which is a traditional differential diagnosis of trichotillomania [2].

Although the clinical diagnosis of many cases of alopecia may be relatively straightforward, often a scalp biopsy is required. However, histopathology of scalp biopsy specimens of patients with scarring or non-scarring alopecia may be of difficult interpretation, particularly when there is not a trustful clinical history as well as adequate tissue sampling and processing [4]. Besides, in longstanding lesions of cicatricial alopecia, the histopathological findings may become less specific, frequently showing only the presence of scar tissue and loss of hair follicles [5].

The gold-standard for a scalp biopsy is a 4-mm punch obtained at the peripheral edge of the patch of alopecia, which may be more representative of the activity of the disease [4]. Some authors defend that two punch biopsies of 4 mm in diameter should be obtained, one from the area of alopecia and the other from the periphery where there is healthy scalp. It should include epidermis, dermis and subcutaneous tissue [5]. Other dermatopathology laboratories suggest a different approach, taking into account the type of alopecia that we are studying, namely, scarring or non-scarring. In scarring alopecias, two punch biopsies should be taken at the periphery of the patch of alopecia, while, in non-scarring alopecias, one biopsy should be from the area of alopecia and the other from an uninvolved area, particularly the occipital region [4].

The specimen is fixed in formaldehyde and embedded in paraffin; thereafter, it is sectioned. The sections can be vertical, transversal or both [4, 5]. In 1984, Headington demonstrated that transverse sections provided excellent histopathological material for morphometric and quantitative study, helping to analyze the hair follicles, the phases of the normal hair growth cycle, and, thereby, to evaluate most types of non-scarring alopecias [5, 6]. Nevertheless, through a transversal analysis, it is difficult to get a perfect representation of the dermoepidermal junction. In turn, vertical sections help to clearly visualize all the layers of the skin, allowing assessment of the dermoepidermal junction, which is particularly useful to study scarring alopecias [4, 5]. However, vertical sections are not useful for quantitative studies on the phases of hair follicles [5]. Because both types of section have advantages and disadvantages, it is recommended to obtain two biopsies, being one for vertical and other for transverse sections [2, 5].

Finally, it is important to point out basic concepts on hair cycle as well as some terms regarding hair biology. Hair follicle cycle is controlled by several mediators, namely, endogenous cytokines, growth factors, hormones and neuropeptides and it starts via catagen (hair follicle involution), followed by a phase of relative hair follicle quiescence (telogen), after which the first anagen (active growth) development is seen, returning back, afterwards, to telogen [7]. About 85% of the hair is in the anagen phase, 1% in the catagen and approximately 10-15% in the telogen phase. Anagen lasts 2-7 years, catagen 2-3 weeks and telogen 100 days [2, 5]. To compare the histologic features among different types of alopecia, terminal to vellus (T/V) ratio is relevant. This is the result of the number of terminal hairs (hair shaft measuring>0.03 mm, greater than the diameter of its inner root sheat) divided by the total of vellus hairs (hair shaft measuring ≤0.03 mm, less than or equal to the diameter of the inner root sheath) at the level of the infundibula. A normal terminal/vellus may range from 5:1 to 7:1 [8].

Since the histopathological findings should always be analyzed in strict correlation with the clinical features, we will start presenting the main clinical differential diagnoses of trichotillomania that may require additional histopathological study, namely alopecia areata, classic pseudopelade of Brocq, syphilitic alopecia, tinea capitis, traction alopecia, trichotemnomania and trichoteiromania, and discuss when histopathology is needed to clarify the diagnosis. Thereafter, we will give account of the main histopathological differential diagnoses of trichotillomania, namely alopecia areata, androgenetic alopecia, congenital temporal triangular alopecia, pressure alopecia and traction alopecia (Table 1).

**Table 1. Clinical and histopathological differential diagnoses of trichotillomania**

| Trichotillomania | |
|---|---|
| Clinical differential diagnoses | Histopathological differential diagnoses |
| Alopecia Areata | Alopecia Areata |
| Classic Pseudopelade of Brocq | Androgenetic Alopecia |
| Congenital Temporal Triangular Alopecia | Congenital Temporal Triangular Alopecia |
| Syphilitic Alopecia | Pressure Alopecia |
| Tinea Capitis | Traction Alopecia |
| Traction Alopecia | |
| Trichotemnomania | |
| Trichoteiromania | |

## 2. TRICHOTILLOMANIA AND CLINICAL DIFFERENTIAL DIAGNOSES

### 2.1. Alopecia Areata

Alopecia areata is a CD8+ T-cell–dependent autoimmune disease and the most frequent type of inflammation-induced hair loss. It can develop during childhood or later and often starts suddenly, most commonly on the scalp and beard. It is characterized by a round patch of hair loss, which typically spreads in a centrifugal or multilocular pattern. Alopecia areata can affect the entire scalp (alopecia areata totalis) and the entire body (alopecia areata universalis) [9, 10]. Trichotillomania can also be found both during childhood and in adults, although more common in children and adolescents. In trichotillomania, other hair-bearing areas of the body can also be affected. The pattern of alopecia may be similar to that of alopecia areata, affecting several and large areas of the scalp, and, then, histopathological examination could be useful to clarify the diagnosis (see section 3). However, typically, the clinical picture is bizarre, with the areas of alopecia having an irregular configuration. We should, however, bear in mind that some patients could also have, at the same time, alopecia areata and trichotillomania [2].

## 2.2. Classic Pseudopelade of Brocq

In 1885, Brocq described a progressive and idiopathic type of alopecia. The alopecic patches would start in the parietal region and they would slowly progress, in a centrifugal direction, throughout several years. However, this entity has been a matter of controversy and discussion, considering the lack of specific clinical and histopathological features. For some authors, this is not a separate entity, but the end-stage of many types of scarring alopecia. Considering that this type of alopecia does not have a specific presentation, it should be included in the clinical differential diagnosis of trichotillomania. Histopathology allows differentiation between both entities, since trichotillomania is a non-scarring alopecia that frequently has characteristic features, while pseudopelade of Brocq is classically considered a form of scarring alopecia, with development of fibrous tracts and loss of folliculosebaceous units [2, 11]. However, other authors have also highlighted that it should not be considered a truly scarring alopecia, but an atrophic variant because elastic fiber network seems to be spared [2].

## 2.3. Congenital Temporal Triangular Alopecia

Congenital temporal triangular alopecia, also called congenital triangular alopecia and temporal triangular alopecia, is a non-scarring type of hair loss that is commonly underdiagnosed. Actually, its clinical presentation may be confused with other types of alopecia, particularly non-scarring types, such as trichotillomania. Although called congenital, it is probably acquired in most patients due to a localized miniaturization of the follicles with unknown etiopathogenesis, leading to regression to vellus hairs [12]. Temporal triangular alopecia usually appears in the first years of life and, sometimes, in adults. Commonly, there is a patch of alopecia in the frontotemporal area; in some cases, other areas can be affected and bilateral patches of alopecia may occasionally be seen [5]. In the setting of difficult clinical differential diagnosis, histopathology could be useful (see section 3).

## 2.4. Syphilitic Alopecia

Syphilis is a "great mimic" and, so, it should be considered in the clinical differential diagnosis of etiologies for alopecia, including trichotillomania.

Syphilitic alopecia is a rare clinical presentation of syphilis. Two types of syphilitic alopecia were described, namely, the symptomatic type, which means that, apart from the alopecia, skin lesions could also be seen on the scalp (commonly, papulosquamous), and the essential type, characterized by hair loss with no other lesions on the scalp [13]. The latter type may be seen as one of three different clinical patterns: moth-eaten or patchy alopecia, diffuse alopecia and mixed pattern, being the moth-eaten pattern of alopecia the most common [13, 14]. Thereby, sometimes, the clinical presentation could raise other clinical differential diagnoses, such as trichotillomania. Serologic screening could be useful to ascertain the diagnosis. The histopathology of syphilitic alopecia may be associated with non-scarring or scarring findings, depending on the duration of the disease. The non-scarring findings can be similar to those of alopecia areata. Furthermore, cases with the moth-eaten pattern show a peribulbar infiltrate composed by lymphocytes and, occasionally, eosinophils and plasma cells, helping to establish the differential diagnosis with trichotillomania. Pigmented casts and trichomalacia are not observed (see section 3) [2].

## 2.5. Tinea Capitis

Tinea capitis is the historic name for dermatophyte infections of the scalp that can also lead to a "moth-eaten" pattern that spreads in a typical ring configuration [15]. The eyebrows and eyelashes can be affected too [11]. The clinical presentation may raise other clinical differential diagnoses, such as trichotillomania. Tinea capitis can be considered the most important dermatophyte infection in children, commonly at the age of five or six years, and it is particularly rare in adults [15]. The most common agents of tinea capitis are the species *Trichophyton* and *Microsporum*. The infection starts through hyphal invasion of the hair follicle and then hyphae grow within the hair shaft. Clinically, this may lead to a more or less severe inflammation depending on the species (respectively, zoophilic or geophilic and anthropophilic) involved [11]. Tinea capitis may be observed with different clinical presentations and six types were described: a gray and scaly patch, where the hair shaft breaks off above the skin surface; a moth-eaten pattern; the black dot pattern, which results from the hair shafts broken off at skin surface; *pityriasis capillitia* pattern, where there is a diffuse scaling of the scalp; pustular type, where yellow pustular lesions are seen; the kerion, which is the most severe, characterized by a deeper infection. When the clinical diagnosis is not clear, the microscopic detection of hyphae through a potassium hydroxide preparation may help to clarify the diagnosis [15]. In histopathology, Periodic Acid-Schiff with diastase stain can show fungal elements (spores and hyphae) in the stratum corneum and within the hair follicles [11].

## 2.6. Traction Alopecia

This is a trauma-induced alopecia and hairstyling is the most common etiology. Although usually seen as a band-like pattern of alopecia in the frontal and temporal areas, sometimes the clinical presentation is not so typical. Depending on the tension forces applied in hairstyling, atypical patterns could be present, leading to consider other clinical differential diagnoses, including trichotillomania [16]. Histopathological findings can be similar to those of trichotillomania (see section 3). Continuous traumatic injury may lead to chronic traction alopecia, resulting in scarring features [2].

## 2.7. Trichotemnomania and Trichoteiromania

Trichotemnomania is an uncommonly reported condition, placed in the obsessive-compulsive spectrum. This disorder means that the patient cuts the hair with scissors or removes the hair by shaving. Another similar condition, also in the obsessive-compulsive spectrum, is trichoteiromania, characterized by hair loss due to repeated rubbing. Clinically, they may resemble alopecia areata, and should be mentioned in the differential clinical diagnoses of trichotillomania. Because the mechanism of removing the hairs is different from trichotillomania, where the mechanism consists of pulling the hair, the histopathology is also different. Both trichotemnomania and trichoteiromania do not have specific histopathologic findings, the hair follicles are normal and there is no inflammation. This helps in the differentiation from trichotillomania and alopecia areata, which usually have associated histopathological features (see section 3) [5, 17].

## 3. Trichotillomania and Histopathological Differential Diagnoses

### 3.1. Trichotillomania

Trichotillomania is a traumatic alopecia and has typical histopathological characteristics, which can help to confirm the diagnosis in most patients. The first two months after the hairs have been pulled represent the best time to perform the biopsy. It is recommended to obtain several sections because only a few of them may exhibit the characteristic features [5]. Through transverse sections, a high percentage of catagen follicles (resulting from changes in hair cycle due to trauma to the hair), pigment casts and traumatized hair follicles could be seen and they have been considered the most relevant findings (Figures 1-4). Minimal or no inflammation is seen. Pigment casts are irregular masses of pigmented cells from the hair matrix, resulting from trauma to the bulbar melanocytes. They are observed in the follicular infundibulum or in the isthmus. The traumatized hair follicles lead to trichomalacia (distortion of the hair), which is another typical finding, but not specific and not always observed. In the early stage of the disease, perifollicular hemorrhage can be seen, helping to establish the diagnosis [2, 5]. Despite the fact that some hair follicles can be distorted due to trauma, the total number of follicles is preserved [11]. A preponderance of catagen and telogen phases can be observed both in trichotillomania and alopecia areata, but another important finding to establish the differential diagnosis is the commonly normal terminal: vellus ratio found in trichotillomania, which may help to distinguish this entity from alopecia areata, its main histopathological differential diagnosis [2]. Finally, as a type of traumatic alopecia, if trichotillomania becomes chronic, scarring features may also be seen [5].

### 3.2. Alopecia Areata

In alopecia areata, there is an abnormal function of hair cycle. The presence of an inflammatory infiltrate is typical, which is an important feature in its distinction from trichotillomania (Figures 5-6). The infiltrate is commonly composed of lymphocytes and Langerhans cells [11]. Eosinophils may also be seen and their presence may exclude androgenetic alopecia and trichotillomania [2]. This inflammation leads to a change in the phase of hair follicles from the anagen to the telogen. This process will be more visible in the late stages of the disease [11, 18]. Furthermore, there is high number of catagen hair follicles, which is the same or relatively higher than that found in trichotillomania [11]. It is important to point out that these findings are related to the duration of the disease. The histopathology in the early stages will not show the preponderance of telogen phase, but only a peribulbar and intrabulbar inflammatory infiltrate will be visible, helping the diagnosis [11, 18]. The peribulbar distribution of the infiltrate is classically compared to a "swarm of bees" [4]. Over time, the number of terminal hairs will be lower and the total of vellus hairs higher. Because the inflammatory infiltrate also involves bulbar melanocytes, melanin incontinence can be observed too [2, 11]. Thereby, pigment casts, a preponderance of catagen phase and trichomalacia could be features of both alopecia areata and trichotillomania. The main difference would be the presence of an inflammatory infiltrate around the bulbs of anagen follicles, which is predominantly lymphocytic and may contain eosinophils [2].

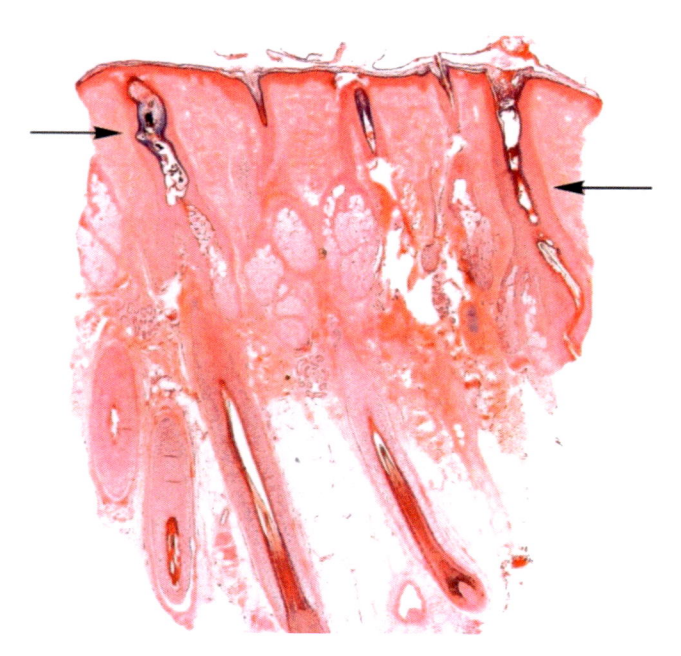

Figure 1. Skin biopsy (hematoxylin and eosin x40) – *Trichotillomania*. Two distorted hair follicles (trichomalacia) and masses of pigmented cells (pigment casts), pointing out the diagnosis of trichotillomania.

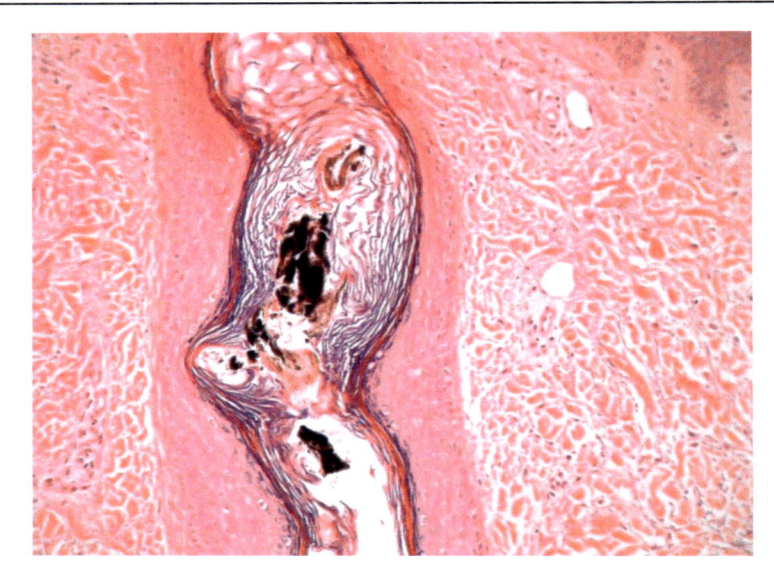

Figure 2. Skin biopsy (hematoxylin and eosin x200) – *Trichotillomania*. The characteristic findings of trichotillomania, pigment casts and trichomalacia, with more detail.

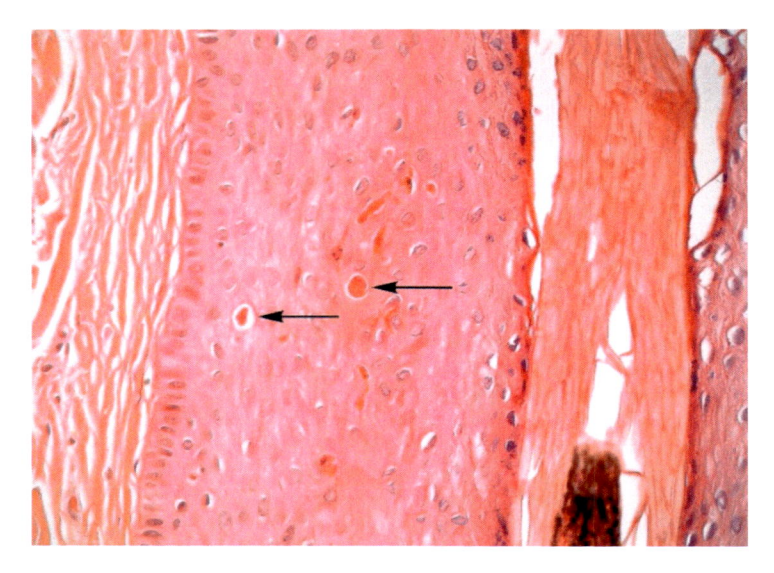

Figure 3. Skin biopsy (hematoxylin and eosin x400) – *Trichotillomania*. Multiple apoptotic keratinocytes in the outer root sheath of the hair follicle, a sign of early catagen phase, a typical finding in trichotillomania.

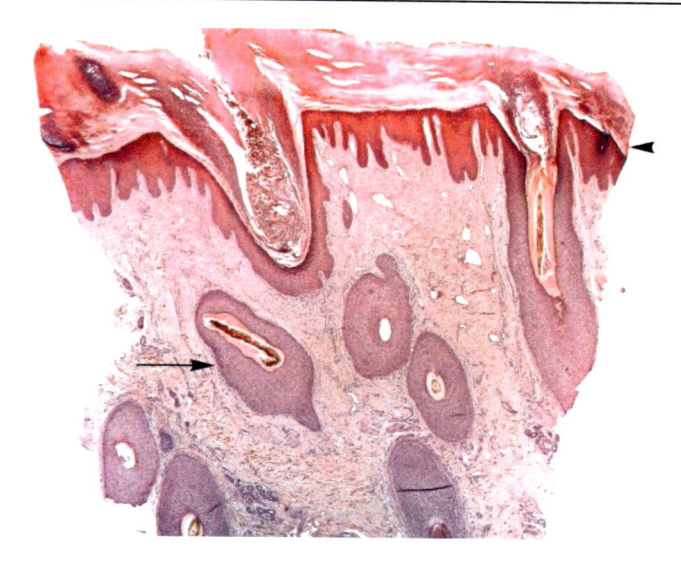

Figure 4. Skin biopsy (hematoxylin and eosin x40) – *Trichotillomania* and *lichenification*. Compact hyperorthokeratosis, hypergranulosis and acanthosis, which can be seen both in trichotillomania and trichoteiromania (arrowhead). Pigment casts and trichomalacia are also present in this biopsy, therefore stating the diagnosis of trichotillomania (arrow).

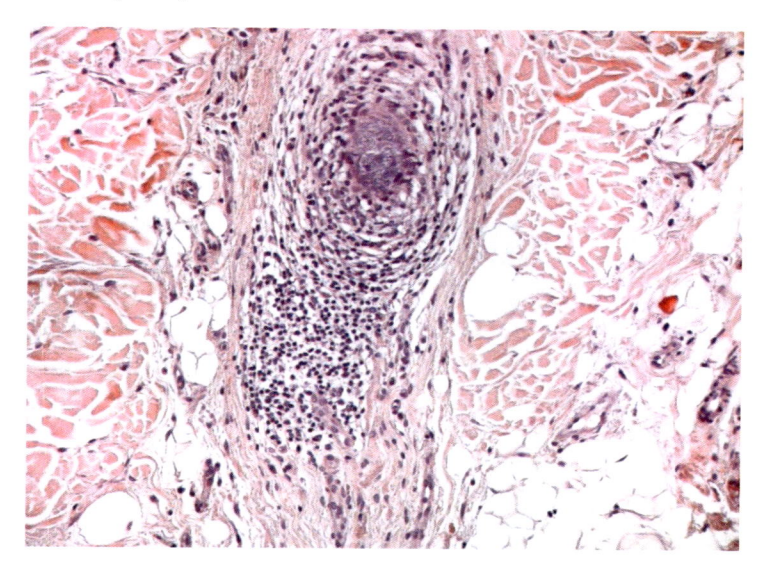

Figure 5. Skin biopsy (hematoxylin and eosin x200) – *Alopecia Areata*. Peribulbar lymphocytes are typical and they are not seen in trichotillomania.

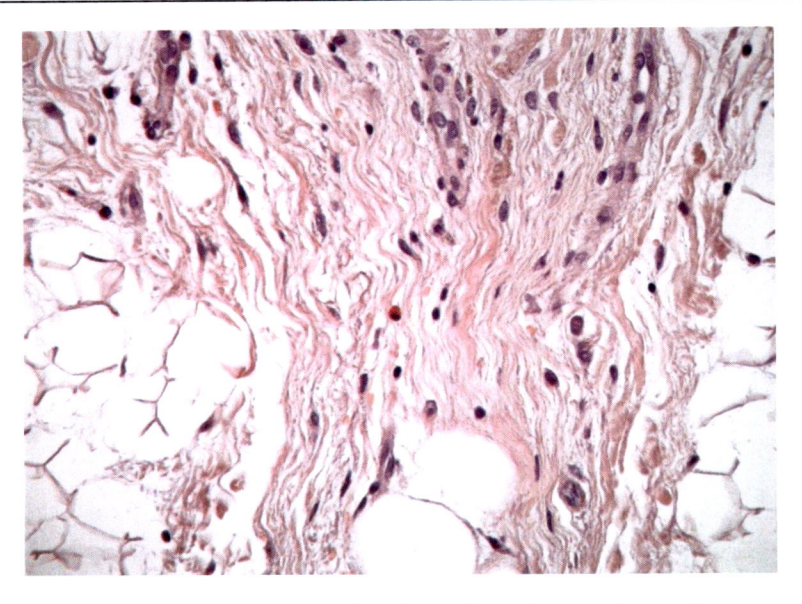

Figure 6. Skin biopsy (hematoxylin and eosin x400) – *Alopecia Areata*. Rare eosinophils can be found around the bulb.

## 3.3. Androgenetic Alopecia

Androgenetic alopecia is considered the most prevalent type of alopecia [10]. Its etiopathogenesis is linked with a genetically conditioned androgen-sensitivity of the hair follicle, leading to particular clinical features and, so, it is not included in the clinical differential diagnosis of trichotillomania [2, 10]. However, it is a type of non-scarring alopecia that, at a histopathological level, has some subtleties that should be distinguished from trichotillomania. There is a reduction of the anagen phase, increasing the number of hair follicles in telogen. However, an increase of catagen hairs is not characteristic of androgenetic alopecia, a finding that is typical of trichotillomania [2]. Furthermore, miniaturization of the hair follicle is not seen in trichotillomania, but it is a characteristic feature of androgenetic alopecia, where there is a reduction in the size of dermal papilla, bulb and hair shaft diameter, increasing the number of vellus hairs. The number of terminal hairs is then reduced but the total number of hairs remains normal. As previously mentioned, these details can be better appreciated through transverse sections [5].

## 3.4. Congenital Temporal Triangular Alopecia

Both trichotillomania and temporal alopecia do not typically have inflammatory infiltrate and the total number of hair follicles is usually normal. However, in temporal alopecia, there is a low number or even total absence of terminal hairs, while in trichotillomania the terminal: vellus ratio is preserved [2]. In addition, trichomalacia and pigment casts are not features of triangular temporal alopecia.

## 3.5. Pressure Alopecia

Pressure alopecia, also called postoperative, is another type of traumatic alopecia. Actually, alopecia resulting from physical trauma can be divided in three types: self-induced alopecia, particularly, trichotillomania; traction alopecia; alopecia that results from accidental trauma [19]. Pressure alopecia is an uncommon type, belonging to the third group. Most of the cases reported were described in the setting of prolonged immobilization and after different surgeries [19, 20]. Thus, the clinical picture is a patch of alopecia over the compressed region of the scalp [11]. It is usually seen in the occipital area [2]. Most of the cases have been explained by local hypoxia affecting hair follicles that usually starts between 3 and 28 days of immobilization and may be transient or permanent [20]. Thereby, at a clinical level, trichotillomania can be easily distinguished considering the following points: there is no recent history of prolonged local pressure in the context of immobilization or surgery; the clinical presentation is bizarre, with one or more patches of incomplete hair loss, with irregular shape, and it is not usually an oval and well-demarcated patch on the occipital region [5, 20]. Therefore, we did not include this entity in the clinical differential diagnoses of trichotillomania. However, at a histopathological level, both are types of traumatic alopecia and should then be compared [20]. Pressure alopecia can have scarring and non-scarring features, depending on the duration of the disease. It may resemble trichotillomania. Pigment casts, catagen and telogen hairs and the absence of inflammatory infiltrate are some of the features that can be shared [2]. However, in pressure alopecia, there are also characteristic histopathologic features: in the early-stages of the disease, intravascular congestion and thrombosis and fat necrosis with foamy macrophages can help to exclude trichotillomania [11, 20].

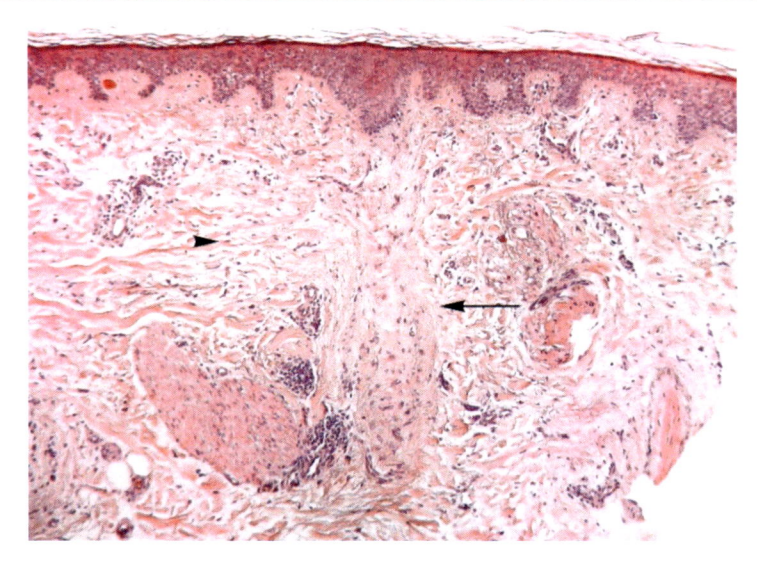

Figure 7. Skin biopsy (hematoxylin and eosin x100) – *Scarring alopecia*. Fibrous tract in the superficial dermis as a result of follicular dropout (arrow), and collagen thickening in the interfollicular dermis (arrowhead), features of late stage disease common to many causes of alopecia. There is only very sparse lymphocytic infiltrate.

## 3.6. Traction Alopecia

The histopathology of traction alopecia shares some features with trichotillomania. This can be easily understood taking into account that both entities are traumatic types of alopecia related to the act of pulling the hair [11]. Nevertheless, the histopathological findings are not as severe as in trichotillomania [5]. As described in trichotillomania, there is no change in the total number of hair follicles and no inflammation. Furthermore, there is a reduction in the number of follicles in the anagen phase, with several catagen and telogen hairs. Similarly to trichotillomania, there is no change in the terminal:vellus hair ratio and pigment casts and trichomalacia can be found, but they are much more uncommon than in trichotillomania. With longstanding traction, these features are lost, developing, in turn, scarring features, with fibrosis around hair follicles. In this stage, the differential diagnosis becomes more difficult and clinical correlation is especially needed (Figure 7) [2, 5, 11].

## CONCLUSION

Trichotillomania is a type of self-induced hair loss, resulting from pulling the hair of the scalp and/or other hair-bearing areas, belonging to the group of traumatic alopecias [19, 21]. It can be observed both in children and adults and a thorough analysis will show regions in the scalp with several hair lengths, a normal hair density and, sometimes, excoriations [21]. However, because the patient may not confess that the alopecia is self-induced and, occasionally, the clinical picture could be untypical or more than one types of alopecia could be present, the clinical diagnosis may become more difficult. For example, trichotillomania affecting the eyebrows and eyelashes can be mistaken for alopecia areata, one of its main differential diagnoses. Furthermore, alopecia areata was reported as a potential trigger for trichotillomania and both conditions can be present at the same time [21]. This finding highlights the psychological impact of hair disorders, their potential connection with psychopathology and the relevance of a holistic approach, provided by psychodermatology, to globally understand and treat the dermatosis, reducing physical distress, diagnosing and treating related anxiety and depression and improving self-esteem [22].

Although histopathology is especially important in the diagnosis of scarring alopecia, it can provide additional information on unexplained cases of non-scarring alopecia as well [23]. Actually, the histopathology of trichotillomania can help to clarify the diagnosis in dubious clinical scenarios. As explained, pigment casts and a high percentage of catagen and telogen hairs as well as perifollicular hemorrhage can help to establish the diagnosis. Typically, there is no inflammation. Trichomalacia can also be a clue the diagnosis, but it is not always present and is also a feature of other conditions, such as alopecia areata [21].

A skin biopsy should be taken from an active region of the scalp, ideally from the periphery. It should go deeply into the hypodermis to see the anagen hair follicles and follow the way of hair growth. Transverse sections give the opportunity to study a high percentage of follicles and, thus, they are especially useful to study trichotillomania and related non-scarring alopecias. Vertical sections are preferable to analyze the total length of the hair follicle. Thereby, to study scarring alopecias, it is recommended to perform both vertical and transverse sections [23]. In the study of trichotillomania, depending on the clinical differential diagnoses established, only transverse sections or both transverse and vertical could be performed.

The purpose of this chapter was to discuss the main clinical differential diagnoses of trichotillomania that might have similar clinical features, requiring additional histopathological study. In Table 2, these diagnoses and the main histopathological differences regarding trichotillomania are summarized. This chapter also intended to discuss the main strictly histopathological differential diagnoses of trichotillomania and a summary of this is presented in Table 3.

**Table 2. Histopathological differential diagnoses of trichotillomania – similarities and differences**

| Trichotillomania | |
|---|---|
| Histopathological differential diagnoses | Main histopathological similarities and differences with Trichotillomania |
| Alopecia Areata | Peribulbar and intrabulbar inflammatory infiltrate (lymphocytes, Langerhans cells, eosinophils); the number of terminal hairs is lower; the total of vellus hairs is higher. |
| Classic Pseudopelade of Brocq | Considered a scarring type of alopecia, with development of fibrous tracts and loss of folliculosebaceous units. |
| Congenital Temporal Alopecia | Low number or total absence of terminal hairs. |
| Syphilitic Alopecia | Similar to alopecia areata; a peribulbar infiltrate of lymphocytes, eosinophils and plasma cells may be seen. |
| Tinea Capitis | Periodic Acid-Schiff with diastase stain can show fungal elements in stratum corneum. |
| Traction Alopecia | Although similar to trichotillomania, histopathology shows less severe findings and a lower percentage of follicles injured. |
| Trichotemnomania | There are no histopathologic changes to report; only hair shaft abnormalities. |
| Trichoteiromania | There are no characteristic histopathologic changes; lichenification and hair shaft abnormalities can be seen. |

**Table 3. Histopathological differential diagnoses of trichotillomania and their main histopathological similarities and differences**

| Trichotillomania | | |
|---|---|---|
| Histopathological differential diagnoses | Similarities with Trichotillomania | Differences with Trichotillomania |
| Alopecia Areata | High number of catagen hair follicles, pigment casts and, sometimes, presence of trichomalacia. | Presence of inflammatory infiltrate; the number of terminal hairs will be lower and the total of vellus hairs higher. |
| Androgenetic Alopecia | The total number of hairs is the same; high number of telogen hairs. | There is not an increase in catagen hairs; higher number of vellus hairs can be observed. |
| Congenital Temporal Alopecia | Absent inflammatory infiltrate; total number of hair follicles is normal. | Low number or total absence of terminal hairs. |
| Pressure Alopecia | Can have scarring and non-scarring features depending on the duration of the disease. Pigment casts, catagen and telogen hairs and absence of inflammatory infiltrate can be observed. | In the early-stages, intravascular congestion and thrombosis as well as fat necrosis with foamy macrophages can be present. |
| Traction Alopecia | Can have scarring and non-scarring features depending on the duration of the disease. No change in the number of hair follicles but a lower number is in the anagen phase, with several catagen and telogen hairs; no inflammation or change in the terminal:vellus hair ratio; pigment casts and trichomalacia can be found. | The findings are less severe. Lower percentage of damaged hair follicles. |

# REFERENCES

[1] Gieler, Uwe, Consoli, Sylvie G., Tomas-Aragones, Lucía, Linder, Dennis M., Jemec, Gregor B. E., Poot, Françoise, Szepietowski, Jacek C, De Korte, J, Taube, Klaus-Michael, Lvov, A., and Consoli, Silla M. 2013. "Self-inflicted lesions in dermatology: terminology and classification–a position paper from the European Society for

Dermatology and Psychiatry (ESDaP)." *Acta dermato-venereologica.* 93(1): 4-12.
[2] Busam, Klaus. 2010. *Dermatopathology.* New York: Elsevier.
[3] Hunt, Nigel, and McHale, Sue. 2005. "The psychological impact of alopecia." *BMJ.* 331:951-953.
[4] Stephanato, Catherine. 2010. "Histopathology of alopecia: a clinicopathological approach to diagnosis." *Histopathology.* 56: 24-38.
[5] Calonje, Eduardo, Brenn, Thomas, Lazar, Alexander J, and McKee, Phillip H. 2011. *McKee's Pathology of the Skin*, 4th Edition. Philadelphia: Elsevier.
[6] Flotte, Thomas J. 2008. "Transverse sectioning of the scalp (Headington technique) in the 19th century." *J. Cutan. Pathol.* 35:82-85.
[7] Paus, Ralf, and Foitzik, Kerstin. 2004. "In search of the "hair cycle clock": a guided tour." *Differentiation.* 72.9-10: 489-511.
[8] Grant-Kels, and Jane M. 2007. *Color atlas of dermatopathology.* New-York: Informa Healthcare.
[9] Gilhar, Amos, Etzioni, Amos, and Paus, Ralf. 2012. "Alopecia Areata." *N. Engl. J. Med.* 366:1515-1525.
[10] Wolff, Hans, Fischer Tobias W, and Blume-Peytavi, Ulrike. 2016. "The diagnosis and treatment of hair and scalp diseases." *Dtsch. Arztebl. Int.* 27;113(21):377-86.
[11] Crowson, A. Neil, Magro, Cynthia M, and Piepkorn, Michael W. 2010. *Dermatopathology.* McGraw-Hill Education/Medical.
[12] Li, Vincent Chum Yin, and Yesudian, Paul Devakar. 2015. "Congenital Triangular Alopecia." *Int. J. Trichology.* 7(2):48-53.
[13] Hernández-Bel, P, Unamuno, B, Sánchez-Carazo, JL, Febrer, I, and Alegre, V. 2013. "Syphilitic alopecia: a report of 5 cases and a review of the literature." *Actas Dermosifiliogr.* 104(6):512-7.
[14] Ye, Yanting, Zhang, Xiaoting, Zhao, Ying, Gong, Yugang, Yang, Jian, Li, Huan, and Zhang, Xingqi. 2014. "The clinical and trichoscopic features of syphilitic alopecia." *J. Dermatol. Case Rep.* 30; 8(3): 78-80.
[15] Nenoff, Pietro, Krüger, Constanze, Schaller, Jörg, Ginter-Hanselmayer, Gabriele, Schulte-Beerbühl, Rudolf, and Tietz, Hans-Jürgen. 2014. "Mycology – an update part 2: dermatomycoses: clinical picture and diagnostics." *J. Dtsch. Dermatol. Ges.* 12(9):749-77.
[16] Barbosa, Aline Blanco, Donati, Aline, Valente, Neusa S, and Romiti, Ricardo. 2015. "Patchy Traction Alopecia Mimicking Areata." *Int. J. Trichology.* 7(4):184-6.

[17] Happle, Rudolf. 2005. "Trichotemnomania: obsessive-compulsive habit of cutting or shaving the hair." *J. Am. Acad. Dermatol.* 52(1):157-9.
[18] Spano, Frank, and Donovan, Jeff C. 2015. "Alopecia areata: Part 1: pathogenesis, diagnosis, and prognosis." *Can. Fam. Physician.* 61(9):751-5.
[19] Ferran, Nicholas A, and Dharmarajah, Rahulan. 2006. "Pressure alopecia following blunt trauma." *Injury Extra.* 37(5): 200-201.
[20] Siah, Tee W, and Sperling, Leonard. 2014. "The histopathologic diagnosis of post-operative alopecia." *J. Cutan. Pathol.* 41(9):699-702.
[21] Sah, Deborah E, Koo, John, and Price, H Vera. 2008. "Trichotillomania." *Dermatol. Ther.* 21(1):13-21.
[22] Jafferany, Mohammad, and França, Katlein. 2016. "Psychodermatology: Basic Concepts." *Acta Derm. Venereol.* 217:35-37.
[23] Mubki, Thamer, Rudnicka, Lidia, Olszewska, Malgorzata, and Shapiro, Jerry. 2014. Evaluation and diagnosis of the hair loss patient: part I. "History and clinical examination." *J. Am. Acad. Dermatol.* 71(3):415.

In: Trichotillomania (Hair Pulling Disorder) ISBN: 978-1-53610-854-5
Editors: K. França and M. Jafferany © 2017 Nova Science Publishers, Inc.

*Chapter 5*

# PHARMACOTHERAPY

## *David Castillo, MD[1],\*, Clinton Enos, MD[2],†, Katlein França, MD, PhD[3,4]‡ and Torello Lotti, MD[3],§*

[1]Department of Dermatology and Cutaneous Surgery
University of Miami Miller School of Medicine, Miami, FL, US
[2]Department of Internal Medicine, Eastern Virginia
Medical School, Norfolk, VA, US
[3] Centro Studi per la Ricerca Multidisciplinare e Rigenerativa,
Università Degli Studi "G. Marconi," Rome, Italy
[4]Department of Dermatology and Cutaneous Surgery,
Department of Psychiatry and Behavioral Sciences,
Institute for Bioethics and Health Policy,
University of Miami Miller School of Medicine, Miami, FL, US

## ABSTRACT

Presently, there is no FDA approved pharmacological treatment for Trichotillomania (TTM). As is the case, multiple drugs and drug classes have been explored for the treatment of TTM, including: antidepressants, antipsychotics, CNS stimulants, and other emerging therapies including *N*-acetyl cysteine (NAC) and nutraceuticals (St. John's wort, milk thistle

---

\* Corresponding author: E-mail: davidecastillos@gmail.com
† Corresponding author: E-mail: enoscw@evms.edu
‡ Corresponding author: E-mail: k.franca@med.miami.edu
§ Corresponding author: E-mail: professor@torellolotti.it

and others). Current evidence suggests that most antidepressants and antipsychotics are not effective in the treatment of TTM, however, there is growing evidence for the use of NAC.

**Keywords:** trichotillomania, hair pulling, obsessive-compulsive disorder, obsessive-compulsive related disorders, skin picking, N-acetylcysteine, St. John's wort, milk thistle, silymarin, myo-inositol, Tricyclic antidepressants, selective serotonin reuptake inhibitors, serotonin-norepinephrine reuptake inhibitors, atypical anti-psychotics

## INTRODUCTION

Currently, there is no pharmacological treatment for TTM that has been approved by the FDA. A variety of pharmacotherapies have been tried, with an emphasis on anti-depressants and anti-psychotics. The association of TTM with obsessive-compulsive spectrum disorder influenced the investigation of anti-depressants and antipsychotics. However, well-designed randomized, placebo-controlled trials are lacking, with the majority of evidence coming from case-reports or trials with inadequate sample size. As such, systematic reviews and meta-analyses have reported equivocal efficacy for these medications. Although there may be a benefit to treating concurrent depression and/or anxiety, many of these medications have serious adverse side effects warranting research in alternative pharmacotherapy. More recently, $N$-acetyl cysteine (NAC) has gained focus with evidence for its use in adults with TTM. The following paragraphs review the evidence for current pharmacological treatment of TTM and the emerging therapy, NAC.

## 1. PHARMACOTHERAPY

### 1.1. Tricyclic Antidepressants

Tricyclic antidepressants (TCAs), named after their chemical structure, block the reuptake of serotonin and norepinephrine in the brain. Originally used as an antidepressant, TCAs have been used in the treatment of several medical disorders, including anxiety and obsessive-compulsive disorder (OCD), but have gained a reputation for their multiple undesired side effects [1]. Swedo et al. performed a double blind, crossover trial comparing clomipramine, which at the time was a new TCA with anti-obsessional effects, and desipramine. Results indicated that clomipramine was affective in the short-term treatment of TTM, however the study was small ($n=13$) and included only women with severe TTM [2]. A more recent study by Ninan et al., further investigated the efficacy of clomipramine in a placebo-controlled trial by comparing cognitive behavior therapy (CBT) with pharmacotherapy (clomipramine) [3]. As evaluated by multiple scoring scales (TTM Severity Scale, TTM Impairment Scale, and the Clinical Global Impressions-Improvement scale), clomipramine induced symptom reduction when compared to placebo, however this result was not found to be statistically significant, nor were the improvement scores, comparable to CBT [3].

## 1.2. Selective Serotonin Reuptake Inhibitors (SSRIs) and Serotonin-Norepinephrine Reuptake Inhibitors (SNRIs)

SSRIs selectively block the reuptake of serotonin in the brain. They are considered first line therapy for depression and a second line therapy for OCD. SNRIs block the reuptake of serotonin and norepinephrine, both of which can have an impact on mood. Fluoxetine, an SSRI used in the treatment of depression, OCD, bulimia nervosa, and panic disorder, has been frequently studied for the treatment of TTM [4-6]. An initial study by Christenson et al., showed no short-term efficacy of fluoxetine in a placebo-controlled crossover study [4]. A subsequent study considered elevated doses of fluoxetine, but again demonstrated no efficacy [5]. Further, a randomized, control trial comparing behavioral therapy, fluoxetine, and no treatment (waiting-list group) revealed no benefit towards treating with fluoxetine [6]. Dougherty et al., in a double-blind, placebo controlled trial, showed that sertraline, an SSRI, as part of dual therapy with habit reversal therapy (HRT) was more efficacious than either treatment alone [7]. Venlafaxine, an SNRI with additional mild effects on dopamine transport, has shown modest efficacy in short-term case series [8]. Reports from a controlled trial approximated the drug to clomipramine and claimed superior results over SSRIs [9].

## 1.3. Atypical Anti-Psychotics

More recently, dopaminergic treatments have been investigated. Olanzapine, a dopamine antagonist, was found to be safe and effective in a randomized, double blind, placebo-controlled trial [10]. A mean dose of 10.8 ± 5.7 mg/day was found effective as measured using the Yale-Brown Obsessive-Compulsive Scale (Y-BOCS) for TTM and the Clinical Global Impressions Severity of Illness scale.

Atypical neuroleptic aripiprazole, a partial dopamine agonist, was initially reported to be effective in a single case report [11], and similar results were found in an open-label trial soon thereafter [12]. Subsequent case reports have reported benefit from treatment with aripiprazole [13, 14], however there is no currently published data from randomized, placebo controlled trials.

## 1.4. Systematic Reviews and Meta-Analyses

Several recent reports have reviewed the treatment options that have undergone formal evaluation for TTM and all have reached, more or less, a common conclusion: Fluoxetine/SSRIs were found to have minimal to no efficacy in the treatment of TTM, and despite the preliminary evidence for olanzapine, clomipramine, no particular medication stands out in efficacy for treatment of TTM [15-18]. These conclusions were made largely due to the fact that many of the above-mentioned studies were single-centered and had a small sample size.

## 1.5. Other Treatments

Naltrexone, an opioid antagonist, showed promising results in a small open-label trial in children [19], however in a subsequent double-blind, placebo controlled trial, naltrexone failed to show a significant reduction in hair pulling as compared to placebo [20]. A preliminary report from a study in a pediatric population with comorbid attention-deficit/hyperactivity disorder (ADHD) demonstrated modest improvement in hair pulling, however this was dependent upon fewer stressful life events per patient [21]. There have also been reports of treating SSRI resistant TTM with the addition of risperidone [22-24], however no formal trials have been published. Other treatments have included: modafinil [25], fenfluramine [26], oxcarbazepine [27], topiramate [28], valproic acid [29], cannabinoid agonists [30], escitalopram [31], citalopram [32], buproprion [33], haloperidol [34], and lithium [35]. There is currently an emerging therapy under investigation, N-acetylcysteine.

## 2. N-ACETYLCYSTEINE

N-acetylcysteine is a derivative of the amino acid cysteine that has been use in the medical practice as antioxidant for several years [36-38]. It is available intravenously, orally and by inhalation [39]. NAC is used for the treatment of many medical illness including acetaminophen overdose, doxorubicin-induced cardiotoxicity, stable angina pectoris, ischemia-reperfusion cardiac injury, acute respiratory distress syndrome, bronchitis, influenza, heavy metal toxicity, chemotherapy-induced toxicity, as a mucolytic for chronic obstructive pulmonary disease, as renal protectant in contrast-induced nephropathy and as a therapeutic agent in the treatment of HIV/AIDS [39, 40]. However, in the current years great effort is being done to study the therapeutic effects of NAC in many psychiatric disorders such as OCD and obsessive-compulsive related disorder (OCRD) (trichotillomania, etc.), autism disorder, bipolar disorder, schizophrenia among others [41].

### 2.1. Pharmacokinetics and Pharmacodynamics

N-acetylcysteine has shown to play an important role in many metabolic pathways in the body, including glutathione generation (antioxidant), modulation of neurotransmitter release, immune-modulation, cell cycle and apoptosis, carcinogenesis and tumor progression, mutagenesis, gene expression and signal transduction, cytoskeleton and cell trafficking and mitochondrial function [39, 42]. Because many psychiatric disorders show dysregulations in these pathways; especially the antioxidant, anti-inflammatory and neurotransmitter modulatory pathways in disorders such as bipolar disorder, major depression and schizophrenia, NAC is being studied for their treatment [43, 44].

#### *2.1.1. Chemistry and Metabolism*
N-acetylcysteine is the N-acetyl derivative of the amino acid cysteine, which is transported in plasma bound to proteins [37, 43]. It is a membrane-permeable substance that passively crosses the cell membrane, once inside the cell it is hydrolyzed to form cysteine, which is the rate limiting substrate of glutathione synthesis [45, 46]. The ability of NAC to cross the blood brain barrier is still controversial [39].

## 2.1.2. Antioxidant Effects

Glutathione (GSH) is the major endogenous antioxidant in the body [44]. Glutathione prevents the oxidative damage caused by radical oxygen species through both non-enzymatic an enzymatic scavenging [46]. This involves a direct reaction and breakdown of reactive oxygen species and an enzyme (GSH peroxidase) mediated destruction of hydrogen peroxide and hydroperoxides [44, 46, 47]. As described previously, NAC is a precursor of cysteine that can be used to replenish the stores of GSH during oxidative stress [43, 48]. Thereby, NAC is essential to maintain an adequate oxidant-antioxidant homeostasis.

Furthermore, NAC has shown intrinsic antioxidant effects by the reaction of the thiol group with hydroxyl radical, OH and hypochlorous acid [39, 44, 49].

## 2.1.3. Immunomodulation

Many psychiatric disorders are associated with alterations in inflammatory pathways [41]. Accordingly, another potential therapeutic benefit of NAC in these disorders are its immunomodulatory properties [37]. NAC is associated to a wide range of anti-inflammatory effects. It has shown to reduce microglia and macrophages activation, reducing the release of cytokines and the induction of oxidative stress damage in the brain [37, 50, 51]. Moreover, NAC has shown to reduce the levels of pro-inflammatory cytokines TNF-$\alpha$, IL-1$\beta$, NF-$\kappa\beta$ and prevention of lipopolysaccharide-related inflammation [39, 44, 52, 53]. These anti-inflammatory actions are thought to be secondary to the upregulation of GSH production, decreasing oxidative stress mediated inflammation [37, 54].

## 2.1.4. Neurotransmitters Modulation

Dysregulation of the glutamatergic system in the brain has shown to be involved in the pathogenesis of obsessive-compulsive and related disorders [55, 56]. NAC acts via activation of the cysteine/glutamate antiporter to increase extrasynaptic glutamate, which in turn activates group II metabotropic glutamate receptors [57]. It is proposed that activation of these receptors regulates the abnormal synaptic release of glutamate [57]. Also, NAC regulates the activation of N-methyl-D-aspartate (NMDA) and 2-amino-3-hydroxy-5-methyl-4-isoxazolepropionate (AMPA) receptors, part of the glutamatergic system [37]. These glutamate modulatory properties may partially explain the therapeutic benefits of NAC in OCRD and other psychiatric conditions.

## 2.1.5. Safety

N-acetylcysteine is widely considered a safe drug with few mild side effects. Deepmala et al. showed in a systematic review of clinical trials about NAC in psychiatry and neurology that the most common reported side effects were gastrointestinal, including abdominal pain or discomfort, heartburn, nausea, vomiting, diarrhea and flatulence. They also reported neurologic adverse effects such as headaches and hand tingling as common [38]. Most side effects occur at high doses (> 3 g/day) and when administered intravenously [44]. In very rare cases, intravenous administration can result in anaphylactic reaction such as urticaria, hypotension, tachycardia, bronchospasm, and angioedema [58-60]. Drug interactions are seen with concomitant administration of NAC and paracetamol, GSH, anticancer drugs and nitroglycerin [46, 48, 61].

Although NAC has been used during pregnancy, more studies are needed to evaluate its safety and thereby should be used with precaution [46].

## 2.2. N-Acetylcysteine for the Treatment of Trichotillomania

Trichotillomania (TTM) is a grooming disorder characterized by recurrent hair pulling which causes significant hair loss and functional impairment classified in the group of obsessive-compulsive and related disorders in the 5th edition of the Diagnostic and Statistical Manual of Mental Disorder from the American Psychiatry Association. As other OCRD, TTM has shown disruption in inflammatory and neurotransmitter pathways (glutamate dysregulation) putting NAC as a promising option for its treatment [41].

N-acetylcysteine has been used for the treatment of TTM and other grooming disorders in the recent decades. There are several case reports and clinical trials supporting the use of NAC in OCRD. Odlaug and Grant reported two cases; a 28-year-old man and a 40-year-old woman that responded to 1800 mg/day of NAC by decreasing hair pulling [62]. Characteristically, when the 28-year-old patient was not compliant with the medication, symptoms returned. Another two cases of a 23 and 19 years old women with TTM were reported to respond to NAC 1.2 g/day [63]. The two women showed complete hair regrowth within 2 and 3 month of treatment, respectively. A few other case reports have also shown benefits with the use of NAC for TMM [64, 65]. There are two randomized control clinical trials (RCT) comparing NAC vs placebo for TTM. The first one was a double blind, controlled clinical trial of NAC in TTM [66]. The study involved 50 adults ranging from 18-65 years of age. Most patients were already on a medication regimen or on psychotherapy. The administered drug dose was 1200 mg/day for 6 weeks followed by 2400 mg/day for 6 more weeks. The study showed that patients on NAC had a significant improvement of TTM symptoms compared to placebo by 9 weeks of treatment. The improvement was measured with the Massachusetts General Hospital Hair Pulling Scale (MGH-HPS) and the Psychiatric Institute Trichotillomania Scale.

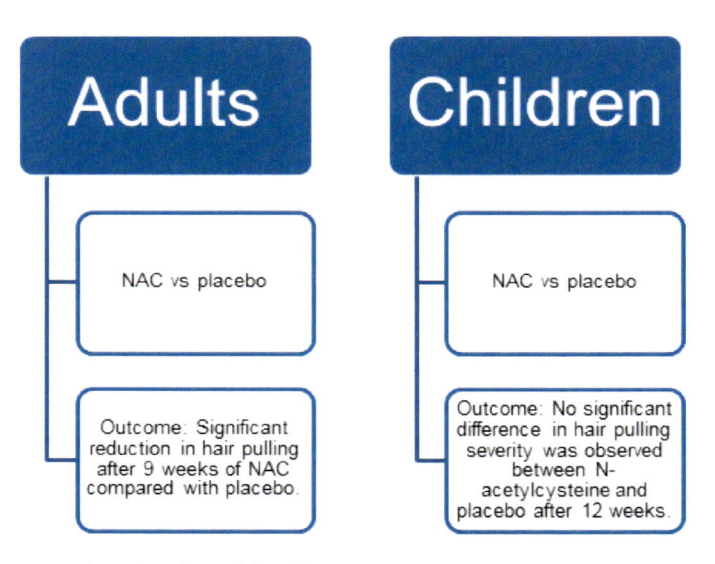

Figure 1. N-acetylcyteine for Trichotillomania, clinical trials in adults vs children [66, 67].

Interestingly, although there is evidence of the effectiveness of NAC in the treatment of TTM in adults, for the pediatric population the evidence is contradictory as shown in figure 1. A double-blinded, placebo-controlled trial was conducted by Bloch et al. to evaluate the use of NAC in TTM in the pediatric population [67]. This study was conducted in 39 patients between 8 to 17 years of age with TTM. Also, patients were already on treatment with a medication regimen and/or behavioral therapy. The study reported no significant improvement or change in severity (primary outcome) measured by the MGH-HPS with the administration of 2400 mg/day of NAC for 12 weeks compare to placebo. According to the authors, the difference between this clinical trial and the previously mentioned could be attributed to the severity of urges pulling which tend to increase with age, and to the fact that children are less aware of the urge symptom.

Even though there is promising evidence of the benefits of NAC in the treatment of TTM in the adult population, due to the mixed results in the two controlled clinical trials done to the date, further research is needed to confirm its effectiveness in the management of TTM [17, 38].

## 2.3. N-Acetylcysteyne for the Treatment of Obsessive-Compulsive and Related Disorders

### 2.3.1. Obsessive-Compulsive Disorder

As described above, obsessive-compulsive and related disorders show abnormalities in many metabolic pathways regulated by NAC. Several clinical trials and case reports have evaluated the use of NAC in these disorders. With respect to OCD, figure 2 describes a RCT that evaluated NAC vs placebo [68]. This study reported a significant gradual decrease in symptoms severity measured by the Y-BOCS in the treatment group compared to placebo. However, case reports results are contradictory. One case reported improvement of symptoms severity measured by the Y-BOCS using NAC 600 mg/day up to 3 g/day in a 58-year-old women with refractory OCD [69]. In contrast, a retrospective case series of six patients with severe, refractory OCD showed that NAC at dose up to 3 g/day was not effective in reducing symptoms. Moreover, only one patient reported improvement of symptoms after 12 weeks of treatment, and two of them experienced worsened symptoms [70].

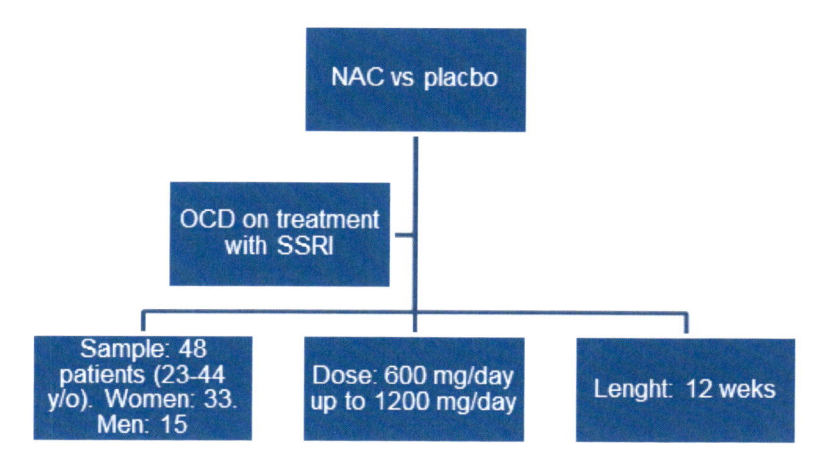

Figure 2. NAC vs placebo for OCD, a randomized clinical trial [68].

In conclusion, the use of NAC in the treatment of OCD seems promising. However, as there is only one controlled clinical trial evaluating it with various study limitations, and case reports are contradictory, further large trials are needed to clarify its effectiveness.

### *2.3.2. Obsessive-Compulsive Related Disorders*

Several case reports and clinical trials are available studying NAC for the treatment OCRD, mainly evaluating pathologic nail biting and excoriation disorder. One case of a 45-year-old woman with both TTM and skin picking disorder was shown to improve with NAC [64]. They reported that after given NAC 1200 mg/day the hair pulling decreased and the skin picking completely resolved. A relapse was seen after discontinuation of the drug, but complete remission of skin picking and improvement of hair pulling was achieved again by restarting NAC, perhaps showing a direct relation between NAC administration and remission of symptoms [64] A few other case reports have shown improvement of skin picking in patients with excoriation disorder on therapy with NAC [62, 71]. An open label prospective case series involving 35 patients (5-39 years of age) with Prader-Willi Syndrome demonstrated a significant decrease in skin picking behavior with 12 weeks of NAC 450-1250 mg/day [72].

Regarding pathologic nail biting, a few cases have been reported to improve this pathologic behavior with NAC therapy [62, 73]. Interestingly, Berk et al. described three women with a significant decreased of nail biting behavior while they were on a clinical trial evaluating NAC in the treatment of bipolar disorder. Also, there is one RCT which evaluated NAC 800 mg/day vs placebo in children and adolescents (6-18 years of age) with chronic nail biting [74]. This study reported a significant increase in nail length at 1 month of treatment. However, this difference was not observed at the second month. Despite the fact that high dropout rate was reported as a significant study limitation, this trial may support that NAC decreases nail biting behavior in children and adolescent in the short term.

Currently, several clinical trials are ongoing to evaluate NAC for the treatment of OCRD [75]. They will aid to determine its relevance in the management of these disorders as many of the studies to date have various limitations and the results are sometimes contradictory. Nevertheless, the evidence supporting the use of NAC for many psychiatric conditions is growing.

## 3. ALTERNATIVE THERAPY FOR OBSESSIVE-COMPULSIVE AND RELATED DISORDERS

The current pharmacological therapy of obsessive-compulsive spectrum disorder is based on antidepressants and antipsychotics, which have failed to prove high response rates and have several adverse effects. In consequence, increasing effort is devoted to find alternative therapies in the recent decades, including natural products (St. John's wort and milk thistle), glycine, myo-inositol (MI), tryptophan, among others [76].

Silymarin is an extract of the herbal antioxidant Milk thistle (Silybum marianum) which contains different flavonoids (silibinin of the most importance) [77]. These flavonoids have shown to modulate the levels of serotonin and dopamine in the central nervous system (CNS) by inhibiting the monoamine oxidase enzyme (MAO), which partially explain its effects on OCRD [76, 78-80]. It also has proven antioxidant effects by attenuating the synthesis of free radicals and nitric oxide [81-83]. One RCT comparing milk thistle vs fluoxetine on patients with OCD showed significant reduction of symptoms using the Y-BOCS by both drugs with no significant difference between them, however this non-inferiority study had a small sample size (n: 35) [84]). More recently, Grant et al. reported 3 patients with obsessive-compulsive and related disorders (OCD, TTM and nail biting) who notably improved by using milk thistle 150 mg once or twice day for a few weeks [85]. Remarkably, when one of the patients stopped milk thistle, nail baiting returned. After restarting the drug, the patient experienced complete remission of the nail biting behavior. This evidence suggests that milk thistle could be effective for the treatment of OCRD, however larger RCTs are needed to support this evidence.

Currently there are two major studies conducted by Taylor and Kobak evaluating St. John's wort (SJW) for the management of OCD. The first was an open label pilot trial on 12 patients with OCD which reported significant improvement of symptoms with SJW [86]. However, the second study, a RCT with sixty patients failed to detect significant difference between SJW and placebo for OCD [87]. Thereby, although further research is needed to clarify these results, SJW is not currently recommended for the treatment of OCD.

Interestingly, current research provides evidence to support the use of MI as monotherapy for obsessive-compulsive and related disorders. A double-blind cross-over study and an open label study of patients with OCD conducted by Fux et al. and Carey et al. respectively, reported significant reduction on Y-BOCS scores when MI 18g/day was used as monotherapy [88, 89]. Further ratifying these results, MI was reported to significantly improve symptoms in three case reports of patients with TTM and skin picking disorder [90]. Although the evidence for MI as monotherapy for obsessive-compulsive and related disorders is remarkable, a few studies failed to report this efficacy when MI was used as augmentation therapy [76, 91, 92].

Despite other nutraceuticals such as glycine and tryptophan might have regulatory effects in CNS pathways involved in the development of obsessive-compulsive and related disorders. There is still few or no clinical evidence about them and more research is needed to recommend them as therapy.

## CONCLUSION

Trichotillomania, commonly called hair-pulling disorder, is a disorder characterized by incontrollable urge of hair pulling causing significant hair loss and functional impairment. Its current treatment is based on psychotherapy and there is no FDA approved pharmacological therapy to date. A number of drugs (SSRIS, SNRs, antipsychotics, etc.) have been studied and are under research for the treatment of TMM and other OCRD. Nevertheless, many of them have failed to be effective or have an unfavorable safety profile. As such, in the recent decades much effort is set on studying alternative therapies, placing special interest on N-acetylcysteine and other nutraceuticals.

The evidence supporting the use of NAC for the management of many psychiatric disorders is growing. Current research highly supports NAC as an effective and very safe option for the treatment of TMM in adults. However, the evidence is contradictory for the pediatric population and further research is needed to clarify this result. Also, other alternative therapies such as silymarin, St. John's wort, myo-inositol among others have been studied showing variable results.

Finally, several clinical trials are ongoing evaluating NAC for TMM and other obsessive-compulsive related disorders to strengthen the preliminary results pointing it out as a promising therapy.

## REFERENCES

[1] Gillman PK. Tricyclic antidepressant pharmacology and therapeutic drug interactions updated. *Br J Pharmacol*. 2007 Jul;151(6):737-48.

[2] Swedo SE, Leonard HL, Rapoport JL, Lenane MC, Goldberger EL, Cheslow DL. A double-blind comparison of clomipramine and desipramine in the treatment of trichotillomania (hair pulling). N Engl J Med. 1989 Aug;321(8):497-501.

[3] Ninan PT, Rothbaum BO, Marsteller FA, Knight BT, Eccard MB. A placebo-controlled trial of cognitive-behavioral therapy and clomipramine in trichotillomania. *J Clin Psychiatry*. 2000 Jan;61(1):47-50.

[4] Christenson GA, Mackenzie TB, Mitchell JE, Callies AL. A placebo-controlled, double-blind crossover study of fluoxetine in trichotillomania. *Am J Psychiatry* [Internet]. 1991 Nov [cited 2016 Aug 08];148(11): 1566-71. Available from: Psychiatry online.

[5] Streichenwein SM, Thornby JI. A long-term, double-blind, placebo-controlled crossover trial of the efficacy of fluoxetine for trichotillomania. *Am J Psychiatry* [Internet]. 1995 Aug [cited 2016 Aug 08];152(8):1192-6. Available from: Psychiatry online.

[6] van Minnen A, Hoogduin KA, Keijsers GP, Hellenbrand I, Hendriks GJ. Treatment of trichotillomania with behavioral therapy or fluoxetine: a randomized, waiting-list controlled study. *Arch Gen Psychiatry*. 2003 March;60(5):517-22.

[7] Dougherty DD, Loh R, Jenike MA, Keuthen NJ. Single modality versus dual modality treatment for trichotillomania: sertraline, behavioral therapy, or both?. *J Clin Psychiatry*. 2006 Jul;67(7):1086-92.

[8] O'Sullivan RL, Keuthen NJ, Rodriguez D, Goodchild P, Christenson GA, Rauch SL, et al. Venlafaxine Treatment of Trichotillomania: An Open Series of Ten Cases. CNS Spectr.1998 Oct;3(9):56–63. doi: 10.1017/S1092852900006519.

[9] Ninan PT, Knight B, Kirk L, Rothbaum BO, Kelsey J, Nemeroff CB. A controlled trial of venlafaxine in trichotillomania: interim phase I results. *Psychopharmacol Bull*. 1998;34(2):221-4.

[10] Van Ameringen M, Mancini C, Patterson B, Bennett M, Oakman J. A randomized, double-blind, placebo-controlled trial of olanzapine in the treatment of trichotillomania. *J Clin Psychiatry* [Internet]. 2010 Oct [cited 2016 Aug 09];71(10):1336-43. Available from: psychiatrist.com

[11] Jefferys D, Burrows G. Reversal of trichotillomania with aripiprazole. *Depress Anxiety*. 2008;25(6):E37-40.

[12] White MP, Koran LM. Open-label trial of aripiprazole in the treatment of trichotillomania. *J Clin Psychopharmacol*. 2011 Aug;31(4):503-6. doi: 10.1097/JCP.0b013e318221b1ba.

[13] Yasui-Furukori N, Kaneko S. The efficacy of low-dose aripiprazole treatment for trichotillomania. *Clin Neuropharmacol*. 2011 Nov-Dec;34(6):258-9.

[14] Sasaki T, Iyo M. Treatment of puberty trichotillomania with low-dose aripiprazole. *Ann Gen Psychiatry.* 2015 Jun;14:18.
[15] Bloch MH, Landeros-Weisenberger A, Dombrowski P, Kelmendi B, Wegner R, Nudel J, et al. Systematic review: pharmacological and behavioral treatment for trichotillomania. *Biol Psychiatry.* 2007 Oct;62(8):839-46.
[16] McGuire JF, Ung D, Selles RR, Rahman O, Lewin AB, Murphy TK, et al. Treating trichotillomania: a meta-analysis of treatment effects and moderators for behavior therapy and serotonin reuptake inhibitors. *J Psychiatr Res.* 2014 Nov;58:76-83.
[17] Rothbart R, Stein DJ. Pharmacotherapy of trichotillomania (hair pulling disorder): an updated systematic review. Expert Opin Pharmacother. 2014 Dec;15(18):2709-19.
[18] Slikboer R, Nedeljkovic M, Bowe SJ, Moulding R. A systematic review and meta-analysis of behaviourally based psychological interventions and pharmacological interventions for trichotillomania. *Clin Psychol* [Internet].2015 [cited 2016 Aug 10]. Available from: Wiley Online Library.
[19] De Sousa A. An open-label pilot study of naltrexone in childhood-onset trichotillomania. *J Child Adolesc Psychopharmacol.* 2008 Feb;18(1):30-3.
[20] Grant JE, Odlaug BL, Schreiber LR, Kim SW. The opiate antagonist, naltrexone, in the treatment of trichotillomania: results of a double-blind, placebo-controlled study. *J Clin Psychopharmacol.* 2014;34(1):134-8.
[21] Golubchik P, Sever J, Weizman A, Zalsman G. Methylphenidate treatment in pediatric patients with attention-deficit/hyperactivity disorder and comorbid trichotillomania: a preliminary report. *Clin Neuropharmacol.* 2011 May-Jun;34(3):108-10.
[22] Gabriel A. A case of resistant trichotillomania treated with risperidone-augmented fluvoxamine. *Can J Psychiatry.* 2001 Apr;46(3):285-6.
[23] Epperson CN, Fasula D, Wasylink S, Price LH, McDougle CJ. Risperidone addition in serotonin reuptake inhibitor-resistant trichotillomania: three cases. *J Child Adolesc Psychopharmacol.* 1999;9(1):43-9.
[24] Senturk V, Tanriverdi N. Resistant trichotillomania and risperidone. *Psychosomatics.* 2002 Sep-Oct;43(5):429-30.
[25] Chamberlain SR, Grant JE, Costa A, Muller U, Sahakian BJ. Effects of acute modafinil on cognition in trichotillomania. *Psychopharmacology* (Berl). 2010 Dec;212(4):597-601.
[26] Mahr G. Fenfluramine and trichotillomania. *Psychosomatics.* 1993 May-Jun;34(3):284.
[27] Leombruni P, Gastaldi F. Oxcarbazepine for the treatment of trichotillomania. *Clin Neuropharmacol.* 2010 Mar-Apr; 33(2):107-8.

[28] Lochner C, Seedat S, Niehaus DJ, Stein DJ. Topiramate in the treatment of trichotillomania: an open-label pilot study. *Int Clin Psychopharmacol.* 2006 Sept;21(5):255-9.
[29] Adewuya EC, Zinser W, Thomas C. Trichotillomania: a case of response to valproic acid. *J Child Adolesc Psychopharmacol.* 2008 Oct;18(5):533-6.
[30] Grant JE, Odlaug BL, Chamberlain SR, Kim SW. Dronabinol, a cannabinoid agonist, reduces hair pulling in trichotillomania: a pilot study. *Psychopharmacology* (Berl). 2011 Dec;218(3):493-502.
[31] Gadde KM, Ryan Wagner H, 2nd, Connor KM, Foust MS. Escitalopram treatment of trichotillomania. *Int Clin Psychopharmacol.* 2007 Jan;22(1):39-42.
[32] Stein DJ, Bouwer C, Maud CM. Use of the selective serotonin reuptake inhibitor citalopram in treatment of trichotillomania. *Eur Arch Psychiatry Clin Neurosci.* 1997;247(4):234–6.
[33] Klipstein KG, Berman L. Bupropion XL for the sustained treatment of trichotillomania. *J Clin Psychopharmacol.* 2012 Apr;32(2):298-9.
[34] Van Ameringen M, Mancini C, Oakman JM, Farvolden P. The potential role of haloperidol in the treatment of trichotillomania. *J Affect Disord.* 1999 Dec;56(2-3):219-26.
[35] Sharma V, Corpse C. Lithium treatment of trichotillomania with comorbid bipolar II disorder. *Arch Womens Ment Health* [Internet]. 2008 Sep [cited 2016 Aug 03];11(4):305-6. Available from: SpringerLink.
[36] LaRowe SD, Mardikian P, Malcolm R, Myrick H, Kalivas P, McFarland K, et al. Safety and tolerability of N-acetylcysteine in cocaine-dependent individuals. *Am J Addict.* 2006 Jan-Feb;15(1):105-10.
[37] Berk M, Malhi GS, Gray LJ, Dean OM. The promise of N-acetylcysteine in neuropsychiatry. *Trends Pharmacol Sci.* 2013 Mar;34(3):167-77.
[38] Deepmala J, Slattery J, Kumar N, Delhey L, Berk M, Dean O, et al. Clinical trials of N-acetylcysteine in psychiatry and neurology: A systematic review. *Neurosci Biobehav Rev* [Internet]. 2015Aug [cited 2016 Aug 20];55:294-321. Available from: ScienceDirect.
[39] Samuni Y, Goldstein S, Dean OM, Berk M. The chemistry and biological activities of N-acetylcysteine. *Biochim Biophys Acta.* 2013 Aug;1830(8):4117-29.
[40] Millea PJ. N-acetylcysteine: multiple clinical applications. *Am Fam Physician.* 2009 Aug;80(3):265-9.
[41] Racz R, Sweet BV, Sohoni P. Oral acetylcysteine for neuropsychiatric disorders. *Am J Health Syst Pharm.* 2015 Jun; 72(11):923-6, 8-9.
[42] Zafarullah M, Li W, Sylvester J, Ahmad M. Molecular mechanisms of N-acetylcysteine actions. *Cell Mol Life Sci.* 2003 Jan;60(1):6-20.

[43] Dodd S, Dean O, Copolov DL, Malhi GS, Berk M. N-acetylcysteine for antioxidant therapy: pharmacology and clinical utility. *Expert Opin Biol Ther* [Internet]. 2008 Nov [cited 2016 Jun 16];8(12):1955-62. Available from: Taylor and Francis Online.

[44] Dean O, Giorlando F, Berk M. N-acetylcysteine in psychiatry: current therapeutic evidence and potential mechanisms of action. *J Psychiatry Neurosci* [Internet]. 2011 Mar [cited 2016 Jun 17];36(2):78-86. Available from: Journal of Psychiatry and Neuroscience.

[45] Sen C. Nutritional biochemistry of cellular glutathione. *J Nutr Biochem.* 1997;8(12):660-72.

[46] Bavarsad Shahripour R, Harrigan MR, Alexandrov AV. N-acetylcysteine (NAC) in neurological disorders: mechanisms of action and therapeutic opportunities. *Brain Behav.* 2014 Mar;4(2):108-22.

[47] Meister A. Glutathione metabolism. *Methods Enzymol.* 1995:251:3-7.

[48] Atkuri KR, Mantovani JJ, Herzenberg LA, Herzenberg LA. N-Acetylcysteine--a safe antidote for cysteine/glutathione deficiency. *Curr Opin Pharmacol* [Internet]. 2007 Jun [cited 2016 Jun 16]7(4):355-9. Available from: ScienceDirect.

[49] Aruoma OI, Halliwell B, Hoey BM, Butler J. The antioxidant action of N-acetylcysteine: its reaction with hydrogen peroxide, hydroxyl radical, superoxide, and hypochlorous acid. *Free Radic Biol Med.* 1989;6(6):593-7.

[50] Masu M, Nakajima Y, Moriyoshi K, Ishii T, Akazawa C, Nakanashi S. Molecular characterization of NMDA and metabotropic glutamate receptors. *Ann N Y Acad Sci.* 1993 Dec;707:153-64.

[51] Rajkowska G, Miguel-Hidalgo JJ. Gliogenesis and glial pathology in depression. CNS Neurol Disord Drug Targets. 2007 Jun;6(3):219-33.

[52] Khan M, Sekhon B, Jatana M, Giri S, Gilg AG, Sekhon C, et al. Administration of N-acetylcysteine after focal cerebral ischemia protects brain and reduces inflammation in a rat model of experimental stroke. *J Neurosci Res.* 2004 May; 76(4):519-27.

[53] Chen G, Shi J, Hu Z, Hang C. Inhibitory effect on cerebral inflammatory response following traumatic brain injury in rats: a potential neuroprotective mechanism of N-acetylcysteine. *Mediators Inflamm* [Internet]. 2008 [cited 2016 Jun 17]. Available from: Hindawi Publishing Corporation.

[54] Kigerl KA, Ankeny DP, Garg SK, Wei P, Guan Z, Lai W, et al. System x(c)(-) regulates microglia and macrophage glutamate excitotoxicity in vivo. *Exp Neurol* [Internet]. 2012 Jan [cited 2016 Jul 02];233(1):333-41. Available from: ScienceDirect.

[55] Chakrabarty K, Bhattacharyya S, Christopher R, Khanna S. Glutamatergic dysfunction in OCD. *Neuropsychopharmacology.* 2005 Sep;30(9):1735-40.

[56] Pittenger C, Bloch MH, Williams K. Glutamate abnormalities in obsessive compulsive disorder: neurobiology, pathophysiology, and treatment. *Pharmacol Ther* [Internet]. 2011 Dec [cited 2016 Jul 02];132(3):314-32. Available from: ScienceDirect.

[57] Moran MM, McFarland K, Melendez RI, Kalivas PW, Seamans JK. Cystine/glutamate exchange regulates metabotropic glutamate receptor presynaptic inhibition of excitatory transmission and vulnerability to cocaine seeking. *J Neurosci* [Internet]. 2005 Jul [cited 2016 Jul 02];25(27):6389-93. Available from: HS Public Access.

[58] Tenenbein M. Hypersensitivity-like reactions to N-acetylcysteine. *Vet Hum Toxicol.* 1984;26 Suppl 2:3-5.

[59] Jones AL, Jarvie DR, Simpson D, Hayes PC, Prescott LF. Pharmacokinetics of N-acetylcysteine are altered in patients with chronic liver disease. *Aliment Pharmacol Ther* [Internet]. 1997 Aug [cited 2016 Jun 17];11(4):787-91. Available from: Wiley Online Library.

[60] Kelly GS. Clinical applications of N-acetylcysteine. *Altern Med Rev.* 1998 Apr;3(2):114-27.

[61] Holdiness MR. Clinical pharmacokinetics of N-acetylcysteine. *Clin Pharmacokinet.* 1991 Feb;20(2):123-34.

[62] Odlaug BL, Grant JE. N-acetyl cysteine in the treatment of grooming disorders. *J Clin Psychopharmacol.* 2007 Apr;27(2):227-9.

[63] Rodrigues-Barata AR, Tosti A, Rodriguez-Pichardo A, Camacho-Martinez F. N-acetylcysteine in the Treatment of Trichotillomania. *Int J Trichology* [Internet]. 2012 Jul-Sep [cited 2016 Jun 25];4(3):176-8. Available from: International Journal of trichology.

[64] Silva-Netto R, Jesus G, Nogueira M, Tavares H. N-acetylcysteine in the treatment of skin-picking disorder. *Rev Bras Psiquiatr.* 2014 Jan-May;36(1):101.

[65] Taylor M, Bhagwandas K. N-acetylcysteine in trichotillomania: a panacea for compulsive skin disorders? *Br J Dermatol* [Internert]. 2014 Nov [cited 2016 Jun 25];171(5):1253-5. Available from: Wiley Online Library.

[66] Grant JE, Odlaug BL, Kim SW. N-acetylcysteine, a glutamate modulator, in the treatment of trichotillomania: a double-blind, placebo-controlled study. *Arch Gen Psychiatry.* 2009 Jul;66(7):756-63.

[67] Bloch MH, Panza KE, Grant JE, Pittenger C, Leckman JF. N-Acetylcysteine in the treatment of pediatric trichotillomania: a randomized, double-blind, placebo-controlled add-on trial. *J Am Acad Child Adolesc Psychiatry.* 2013 Mar;52(3):231-40.

[68] Afshar H, Roohafza H, Mohammad-Beigi H, Haghighi M, Jahangard L, Shokouh P, et al. N-acetylcysteine add-on treatment in refractory obsessive-compulsive disorder: a randomized, double-blind, placebo-controlled trial. *J Clin Psychopharmacol.* 2012 Dec;32(6):797-803.

[69] Lafleur DL, Pittenger C, Kelmendi B, Gardner T, Wasylink S, Malison RT, et al. N-acetylcysteine augmentation in serotonin reuptake inhibitor refractory obsessive-compulsive disorder. *Psychopharmacology* (Berl) [Internet]. 2005 Dec [cited 2016 Jul 02];184(2):254-6. Available from: SpringerLink.

[70] Van Ameringen M, Patterson B, Simpson W, J. T. N-acetylcysteine augmentation in treatment resistant obsessive compulsive disorder: A case series. *J Obsessive Compuls Relat Disord* [Internet]. 2013 [cited 2016 Jul 02];2(1):48-52. Available from: ScienceDirect.

[71] Grant JE, Odlaug BL, Chamberlain SR, Keuthen NJ, Lochner C, Stein DJ. Skin picking disorder. *Am J Psychiatry*. 2012 Nov;169(11):1143-9.

[72] Miller JL, Angulo M. An open-label pilot study of N-acetylcysteine for skin-picking in Prader-Willi syndrome. *Am J Med Genet A* [Internet]. 2013 Dec [cited 2016 Jul 05];164A(2):421-4. Available from: Wiley Online Library.

[73] Berk M, Jeavons S, Dean OM, Dodd S, Moss K, Gama CS, et al. Nail-biting stuff? The effect of N-acetyl cysteine on nail-biting. *CNS Spectr*. 2009 Jul;14(7):357-60.

[74] Ghanizadeh A, Derakhshan N, Berk M. N-acetylcysteine versus placebo for treating nail biting, a double blind randomized placebo controlled clinical trial. *Antiinflamm Antiallergy Agents Med Chem*. 2013;12(3):223-8.

[75] Oliver G, Dean O, Camfield D, Blair-West S, Ng C, Berk M, et al. N-acetyl cysteine in the treatment of obsessive compulsive and related disorders: a systematic review. *Clin Psychopharmacol Neurosci*. 2015 Apr;13(1):12-24.

[76] Camfield DA, Sarris J, Berk M. Nutraceuticals in the treatment of obsessive compulsive disorder (OCD): a review of mechanistic and clinical evidence. *Prog Neuropsychopharmacol Biol Psychiatry* [Internet]. 2011 Feb [cited 2016 Jul 05];35(4):887-95. Available from: ScienceDirect.

[77] Surai PF. Silymarin as a Natural Antioxidant: An Overview of the Current Evidence and Perspectives. *Antioxidants (Basel)* [Internet]. 2015 March [cited 2016 Jul 16];4(1):204-47. Available from: Antioxidants.

[78] Mazzio EA, Harris N, Soliman KF. Food constituents attenuate monoamine oxidase activity and peroxide levels in C6 astrocyte cells. *Planta Med*. 1998 Oct;64(7):603-6.

[79] Osuchowski MF, Johnson VJ, He Q, Sharma RP. Alterations in regional brain neurotransmitters by silymarin, a natural antioxidant flavonoid mixture, in BALB/ c mice. *Pharm Biol*. 2004;42(4-5):384–9.

[80] Lu P, Mamiya T, Lu L, Mouri A, Niwa M, Kim HC, et al. Silibinin attenuates cognitive deficits and decreases of dopamine and serotonin

induced by repeated methamphetamine treatment. *Behav Brain Res.* 2010 March;207(2):387-93.

[81] Zhu HJ, Brinda BJ, Chavin KD, Bernstein HJ, Patrick KS, Markowitz JS. An assessment of pharmacokinetics and antioxidant activity of free silymarin flavonolignans in healthy volunteers: a dose escalation study. *Drug Metab Dispos* [Internet]. 2013 Jul [cited 2016 Jul 16];41(9):1679-85. Available from: ASPET.

[82] Schrieber S, J., Hawke RL, Wen Z, Smith pc, Reddy KR, Wahed AS, et al. Differences in the disposition of silymarin between patients with nonalcoholic fatty liver disease and chronic hepatitis c. *Drug Metab Dispos* [Internet]. 2011 Aug [cited 2016 Aug 01];39(12):2182–90. Available from: ASPET.

[83] Calani L, Brighenti F, Bruni R, Del Rio D. Absorption and metabolism of milk thistle flavanolignans in humans. *Phytomedicine* [Internet]. 2012 Oct [cited 2016 Aug 01];20(1):40-6. Available from: ScienceDirect.

[84] Sayyah M, Boostani H, Pakseresht S, Malayeri A. Comparison of Silybum marianum (L.) Gaertn. with fluoxetine in the treatment of Obsessive-Compulsive Disorder. *Prog Neuropsychopharmacol Biol Psychiatry* [Internet]. 2009 Dec [cited 2016 Jul 16];34(2):362-5. Available from: ScienceDirect.

[85] Grant JE, Odlaug BL. Silymarin treatment of obsessive-compulsive spectrum disorders. *J Clin Psychopharmacol.* 2015 Jun;35(3):340-2.

[86] Taylor LH, Kobak KA. An open-label trial of St. John's Wort (Hypericum perforatum) in obsessive-compulsive disorder. *J Clin Psychiatry.* 2000 Aug;61(8):575-8.

[87] Kobak KA, Taylor LV, Bystritsky A, Kohlenberg CJ, Greist JH, Tucker P, et al. St John's wort versus placebo in obsessive-compulsive disorder: results from a double-blind study. *Int Clin Psychopharmacol.* 2005 Nov;20(6):299-304.

[88] Fux M, Levine J, Aviv A, Belmaker RH. Inositol treatment of obsessive-compulsive disorder. *Am J Psychiatry.* 1996 Sep;153(9):1219-21.

[89] Carey PD, Warwick J, Harvey BH, Stein DJ, Seedat S. Single photon emission computed tomography (SPECT) in obsessive-compulsive disorder before and after treatment with inositol. *Metab Brain Dis.* 2004;19(1-2):125-34.

[90] Seedat S, Stein DJ, Harvey BH. Inositol in the treatment of trichotillomania and compulsive skin picking. *J Clin Psychiatry.* 2001 Jan;62(1):60-1.

[91] Fux M, Benjamin J, Belmaker RH. Inositol versus placebo augmentation of serotonin reuptake inhibitors in the treatment of obsessive-compulsive disorder: a double-blind cross-over study. *Int J Neuropsychopharmacol.* 1999 Sep;2(3):193-5.

[92] Seedat S, Stein DJ. Inositol augmentation of serotonin reuptake inhibitors in treatment-refractory obsessive-compulsive disorder: an open trial. *Int Clin Psychopharmacol.* 1999 Nov;14(6):353-6.

In: Trichotillomania (Hair Pulling Disorder)　　ISBN: 978-1-53610-854-5
Editors: K. França and M. Jafferany　　© 2017 Nova Science Publishers, Inc.

*Chapter 6*

# NON-PHARMACOLOGICAL TREATMENTS FOR TRICHOTILLOMANIA

## *Philip D. Shenefelt, MD*
Department of Dermatology and Cutaneous Surgery
University of South Florida, College of Medicine, Tampa, FL, US

### ABSTRACT

Trichotillomania is a repetitive hair manipulating and pulling habit disorder that leads to hair breakage and hair extraction with temporary alopecia. Sometimes patients deny any involvement in the process. Hair itself is composed of dead keratin except at the root bulb. Repeated twisting fractures the hair shaft with breakage, while pulling extracts the entire hair including the root bulb. Non-pharmacological treatments for trichotillomania involve various approaches to alter the self-destructive dysfunctional habit patterns of hair pulling. Methods include insight-oriented psychoanalysis, Cognitive-Behavioral Therapy (CBT) including Habit Reversal Training (HRT), Acceptance and Commitment Therapy (ACT), Dialectic Behavioral Therapy (DBT), hypnotic suggestion, and psychosomatic hypnoanalysis.

## PSYCHOANALYSIS

Psychoanalysis has become economically less viable as a current non-pharmacological treatment method due to its lengthy slow treatment process and changing reimbursement patterns. It does however provide an interesting historical perspective and viewpoint regarding trichotillomania. Koblenzer (1999) summarized psychoanalytic thought with respect to hair and hair pulling. Hair visibility makes it readily available as a medium for representation of emotional content. As an infant, the tactile and visual experience of the mother's skin and hair are important bonding factors during imprinting or attachment. As a toddler, unresolved conflict and emotional issues often arise during toilet training with the struggle for self-assertion. The preschool child solidifies gender identification and attraction toward the parent of the opposite sex creating more unresolved conflict. The elementary school aged child learns to interact with the peer group and deal with reality, again often creating more unresolved unconscious conflict. Adolescence has its hormonal upheaval and burgeoning sexual desires counterbalanced by social compliance with its innate unconscious conflicts. Hair can represent virility on a man and beauty on a woman and has sexual connotations. Skin and hair can be used symbolically to express unconscious ideas, desires, and conflicts. In some individuals, hair twisting to the point of hair breakage and hair pulling to the point of extracting hairs can become a habit designed to relieve anxiety or tension generated by unresolved unconscious conflict. There are elements of impulse control disorder and obsessive-compulsive disorder (OCD) involved in hair pulling. Hair may substitute for the mother as a transitional object. Parenting issues are often involved in patients with trichotillomania, especially ambivalent or non-empathetic or non-nurturing mother-child relationships, particularly during the oral-tactile phase prior to 18 months old. Anger often plays a role in the self-destructive hair pulling. Koblenzer (1999) presented a case of a 14 year old girl who had been pulling out eyelashes and eyebrows since age 10. Behavior therapy had failed to stop the hair pulling. She had been weaned from breast to bottle at 3 months old and used thumb sucking as a transitional object. An angry and willful child, she was displaced from her crib at age 2 at the height of her anal phase by the birth of a brother. She then began nail biting as well as continuing thumb sucking and kept her parents up at night by fussing. At age 10 it was found that her vigorous thumb sucking had pushed her front teeth out of alignment requiring braces and cessation of thumb sucking. It was at that point that she began pulling out her eyebrow and eyelash hairs. Her mother was described as narcissistic and resentful of the restrictions imposed upon her by the needs of her children. Her father had restricted emotional range and worked long hours out of the house to avoid the emotional tension at home. The patient was treated with insight-oriented psychotherapy once weekly over the course of 2 years with resolution of the trichotillomania. She worked through her anger and guilt feelings with respect to her mother and experienced re-parenting through her therapist. Koblenzer had previously presented a case series of using psychoanalysis with resolution of trichotillomania in 4 of 6 patients at a medical meeting in 1989.

## COGNITIVE-BEHAVIORAL THERAPY (CBT)

Cognitive-behavioral therapy (CBT) methods help to alter dysfunctional thought patterns (cognitive) or actions (behavioral) that damage the hair through twisting or pulling. These methods include habit reversal training (HRT) (Azrin and Nunn 1973). Patients learn competing reaction training such as stiffening the elbows and clenching the fists rather than hair pulling. They also have awareness of hair pulling training, identifying response precursors such as hair touching, identifying habit-prone situations, relaxation training, prevention training, habit interruption, positive hair care, competing reaction practice, self-recording or hair pulling, display of improvement practicing their competing movement, social support enlistment, and annoyance review to identify all problems created by the hair pulling. Azrin et al. (1980) in a randomized trial compared habit reversal training (HRT) with negative practice. Habit reversal produced about a 90% hair pulling reduction compared with negative practice hair pulling reduction of 68% after 3 months. Rothbaum and Ninan (1999) published a manual for cognitive-behavioral treatment of trichotillomania. Session 1 involves information gathering, session 2 habit reversal training, sessions 3 and 4 coping skills with muscle relaxation and breathing control, session 5 thought stopping, session 6 cognitive restructuring, session 7 guided self-dialogue, session 8 role playing and covert modeling, and session 9 relapse prevention. Gupta and Gargi (2012) reported successful treatment of trichotillomania using habit reversal training with stimulus control and self-monitoring. The Massachusetts General Hospital Hair Pulling Scale (MGH-HPS) (Keuthen et al. 1995) was applied to access severity and progress of the patient over 12 sessions, starting at 22 and becoming 0 by session 6 and remaining negative thereafter. Other rating scales employed include the National Institute of Mental Health Trichotillomania

Scales (Swedo et al. 1989) and the Psychiatric Institute Trichotillomania Scale (Winchel et al. 1992).

McGuire et al. (2014) performed a meta-analysis of randomized control trials using behavior therapy to treat trichotillomania and found a significant pooled effect size for behavior therapy compared with controls. A randomized control trial comparing cognitive therapy to behavior therapy (Keijsers et al. 2016) failed to show a significant difference between cognitive therapy and behavior therapy. Franklin et al. (2011) conducted a randomized control trial for pediatric trichotillomania of behavior therapy compared with minimal attention controls. The behavior therapy patients received 8 weeks of active treatment followed by a maintenance treatment phase of 4 visits over 8 weeks. Trichotillomania scores were significantly lower for the behavior therapy group by 8 weeks compared with the minimal attention controls. Toledo et al. (2015) conducted randomized group cognitive-behavioral treatment for trichotillomania versus supportive therapy and found significant improvement in the group cognitive-behavioral therapy subjects compared with the supportive therapy subjects. Movement decoupling (Moritz and Rufer 2011) is a self-help technique where movement of the arm toward the hair is redirected toward another body part or toward a certain point in the room with an accelerated movement. After two weeks, the decoupled motion can be altered to less stereotypic. Patients were to practice at least 15 minutes daily to reshape the habit. The MGH-HPS was administered along with the Beck Depression Inventory (BDI) to randomized patients in which a decoupled motion group was compared with a progressive muscle relaxation group. The decoupled motion group had significant improvement both in the MGH-HPS and the BDI, while the progressive muscle relaxation group showed no significant change in either MGH-HPS or BDI. An internet-based self-help randomized control trial comparing decoupling and progressive muscle relaxation (Weidt et al. 2015) showed some relative improvement in the decoupled motion group compared with the progressive muscle relaxation group, but the difference did not reach a level of significance in the internet-based study.

## ACCEPTANCE AND COMMITMENT THERAPY (ACT)

Acceptance and commitment therapy (ACT) focuses on changing the response to the patient's own thinking and feelings by directing the patient toward acceptance of their emotions and life experiences and to have the patient be present in the face of strong emotion that they might otherwise be avoiding (Montgomery et al. 2011). Woods et al. (2006) utilized ACT and habit reversal for trichotillomania in a randomized control trial comparing ACT and habit reversal to those on a waiting list. There was significantly greater response at 66% in the treatment group compared with 8% response in the waiting list group. Treatment effect was generally maintained at a 3 month follow-up. Greater treatment compliance was found to predict a favorable clinical response.

## DIALECTICAL BEHAVIORAL THERAPY (DBT)

Dialectical behavioral therapy (DBT) was originally developed for suicidal emotionally dysregulated patients with borderline personality disorder (MacPherson et al. 2013). DBT incorporates aspects of behavioral approaches, dialectical philosophy emphasizing the existence of simultaneous opposing forces (thesis and antithesis), and dialectical change produced from the recognition of opposing forces with validity at each pole transitioning into a synthesis incorporating Zen practice. The goal is to reduce polarized thoughts and behaviors. Randomized control trials have shown significant improvements using DBT to help reduce problem behaviors. Keuthen et al. (2102) conducted a randomized control trial of DBT-enhanced cognitive-behavioral treatment for trichotillomania with 11 weeks of acute treatment and 3 months of maintenance treatment and found significant improvement in hair pulling reduction and emotional regulation compared with minimal attention controls. Welch and Kim (2012) applied DBT to trichotillomania with 16 weeks of individual DBT along with trichotillomania psychoeducation, habit reversal, and stimulus control. There was significant improvement in hair pulling, emotional regulation, anxiety, and depression post treatment.

## Hypnotic Suggestion

Hypnosis involves utilization of the natural trance state to facilitate coordination and cooperation of conscious wishes and willpower with unconscious habits and desires and conflicts. The hypnotic trance involves narrowed and focused attention and increased suggestibility and receptivity. If the patient is already in trance, that may be utilized, and if not, trance may be induced. There is a natural genetic predisposition that permits some individuals to shift into trance more readily than others (Szekely et al. 2010). Hypnotic suggestion can facilitate habit pattern change. It often takes 20 or more repetitions to change a habit, so teaching self-hypnosis followed by having the patient do hypnotic homework is important in obtaining results. Fabbri and Dy (1974) successfully used hypnotic treatment of trichotillomania in two cases and ascribed its effectiveness to anxiety suppression and habit substitution. Galski (1981) used hypnotic suggestion successfully in a 26 year old woman to promote awareness of reaching toward the scalp, to increase the sensitivity of the scalp to hair pulling, and to immediately become aware and let go of the hair and relax as a new habit. Hall and McGill (1986) used hypnobehavioral treatment to successfully eliminate both trichotillomania and bulimia in a 22 year old woman. Barabasz (1987) used hypnotic suggestion enhanced by restricted environmental stimulation technique (REST) with posthypnotic suggestions for increased awareness of hair pulling, self-control, and choice in hair pulling in a small case series. All 4 patients in the study stopped hair pulling, and at one year three of the four had maintained recovery while one had relapsed. Zalsman et al. (2001) used hypnotherapy for trichotillomania in three adolescents who became protective patrons of their weak and vulnerable hairs with cessation of hair pulling. Iglesias (2003) used hypnosis in three children ages 8, 10, and 11 years old that with parental approval redefined the patient's hair as their own property and affirmed their sole responsibility for care and maintenance of the hair. This choice and self-agency was sufficient along with hypnotic ego strengthening suggestions to end the hair pulling in each case. Dr. Dabney Ewin (personal communication) has had moderately good results in three cases with disrupting the unconscious activity with the suggestion to "Let it be impossible to raise your hand above the shoulder towards your hair without first stopping to look at your hand and make a conscious decision about possibly doing something different with your hand." He would have to reinforce that suggestion about every six months, but if he could get an ideomotor confirmation that the idea was agreeable, it would last for increasingly longer times.

## Psychosomatic Hypnoanalysis

A history of increased psychological traumatic life events mostly occurring in childhood has been reported (Ozten et al. 2015) averaging 4 per person for trichotillomania patients compared with 2.5 per person for normal controls. Rowen (1981) used hypnotic age regression to look for unconscious causes of the 21 year old patient's hair pulling habit. In trance he recalled that he began pulling out hairs at age 7 to help relieve stress generated in response to his hostile father. By age 10 he got a peculiar pleasurable feeling from pulling a hair. He was again hypnotically regressed to age 7 and the suggestion was made that he experience discomfort when pulling a hair and that the discomfort would progressively increase as his age was progressed year by year until his present age of 21. He ceased pulling hairs and remained free of trichotillomania upon follow-up 6 months later. Hypnoanalysis with ideomotor signaling had been used successfully to obtain responses in 3 cases of psychogenic excoriations where hypnotic direct suggestion had failed (Iglesias 2005). Psychosomatic hypnoanalysis (Shenefelt 2016) means that the somatic bridge hypnotic regression to first occurrence of trichotillomania involving hair pulling is used, followed by exploration using LeCron's (1961) seven key factors as further described by Ewin and Eimer (2006). The seven most common factors causing emotional difficulties and illnesses are Conflict, Organ language (in this case hair pulling—"I wanted to pull my hair out!"), Motivation or secondary gain, Past traumatic experiences, Active identification with a parent or other figure, Self-punishment, and Suggestion or imprint to pull hair, with the mnemonic C.O.M.P.A.S.S. Neutralizing suggestions can then help to inactivate the highly charged negative emotion connected to the traumatic memory. This technique can be used for screening for psychosomatic factors related to triggering or exacerbating hair pulling. Individuals that have not responded to direct posthypnotic suggestion to cease pulling hair may have psychological blockages that can be explored and corrected through psychosomatic hypnoanalysis.

## REFERENCES

Azrin NH, Nunn RG. Habit-reversal: a method of eliminating nervous habits and tics. *Behav Res Ther*. 1973; 11:141–149.

Azrin NH, Nunn RG, Frantz SE. Treatment of hairpulling (trichotillomania): a comparative study of habit reversal and negative practice training. 1980; *J Behav Ther Exp Psychiatry* 11:13-20.

Barabasz M. (1987) Trichotillomania: a new treatment. *Int J Clin Exper Hypn* 1987; 35:3, 146-154.

Ewin D, Eimer BNM. Ideomotor Signals for Rapid Hypnoanalysis: a How-to Manual. Springfield, Illinois: Charles C Thomas, Publishers, 2006.

Fabbri R, Dy AJ. Hypnotic treatment of trichotillomania: two cases, *Int J Clin Exper Hypn* 1974; 22(3): 210-215.

Franklin ME, Edson AL, Ledley DA, Cahill SP. Behavior therapy for pediatric trichotillomania: a randomized controlled trial. *J Am Acad Child Adolesc Psychiatry.* 2011; 50:763–771.

Galski TJ. The adjunctive use of hypnosis in the treatment of trichotillomania: a case report. *Am J Clin Hypn* 1981; 23(3): 198-201.

Gupta S, Gargi PD. Habit reversal training for trichotillomania. *Int J Trichol.* 2012; 4: 39-41.

Hall JR, McGill JC. Hypnobehavioral treatment of self-destructive behavior: trichotillomania and bulimia in the same patient, *Am J Clin Hypn.* 1986; 29:1, 39-46.

Iglesias A. Three failures of direct suggestion in psychogenic dermatitis followed by successful intervention. *Am J Clin Hypn.* 2005; 47(3):191-198.

Iglesias A. Hypnosis as a vehicle for choice and self-agency in the treatment of children with trichotillomania, *Am J Clin Hypn* 2003; 46:(2): 129-137.

Keijsers GPJ, Maas J, van Opdorp A, van Minnen A. Addressing self-control cognitions in the treatment of trichotillomania: a randomized controlled trial comparing cognitive therapy to behaviour therapy. *Cogn Ther Res* 2016; 40:522–531.

Keuthen NJ, O'Sullivan RL, Ricciardi JN, Shera D, Savage CR, Borgmann AS, Jenike MA, Baer L. The Massachusetts General Hospital (MGH) hairpulling scale, 1: development and factor analysis. *Psychother Psychosomat* 1995; 64: 141-145.

Keuthen NJ, Rothbaum BO, Fama J, Altenburger E, Falkenstein MJ, Sprich SE, Kearns M, Meunier S, Jenike MA, Welch SS. DBT-enhanced cognitive-behavioral treatment for trichotillomania: a randomized controlled trial. *J Behav Addict.* 2012; 1:106–114.

Koblenzer CS. Psychoanalytic perspectives on trichotillomania. In: Stein DJ, Christenson G, Hollander E, editors. Trichotillomania. Washington, DC: American Psychiatric Press; 1999:125–145.

LeCron LM. Techniques of Hypnotherapy. New York, New York, Julius Publishers 1961.

MacPherson HA, Cheavens JS, Fristad MA. Dialectical Behavior Therapy for Adolescents: *Theory, Treatment Adaptations, and Empirical Outcomes Clin Child Fam Psychol Rev.* 2013; 16:59–80.

McGuire JF, Ung D, Selles RR, Rahman O, Lewin AB, Murphy TK, Storch EA. Treating trichotillomania: a meta-analysis of treatment effects and moderators for behavior therapy and serotonin reuptake inhibitors. *J Psychiatr Res.* 2014; XX0: 76–83.

Montgomery KL, Kim JS, Franklin C. Acceptance and commitment therapy for psychological and physiological illnesses: a systemic review for social workers. *Health Social Work* 2011; 16(3): 169-181.

Moritz S, Rufer M. Movement decoupling: A self-help intervention for the treatment of trichotillomania. *J. Behav. Ther. And Exp. Psychiat.* 2011; 42: 74-80.

Özten E, Sayar GH, Eryılmaz G, Kagan G, Işık S, Karamustafalıoglu O. The relationship of psychological trauma with trichotillomania and skin picking. *Neuropsychiatric Disease and Treatment* 2015; 11: 1203–1210.

Rothbaum BO, Ninan PT. Manual for the cognitive-behavioral treatment of trichotillomania. In: Stein DJ, Christenson GA, Hollander E, editors. Trichotillomania. Washington, DC, USA: American Psychiatric Press; 1999: 263-284.

Rowen R. Hypnotic age regression in the treatment of a self-destructive habit: trichotillomania. *Am J Clin Hypn* 1981; 23(3): 195-197.

Shenefelt PD. Skin Disorders. In Elkins GR, Clinician's Guide to Medical and Psychological Hypnosis: Foundations, Applications, and Professional Issues. New York, New York, Springer Publishing 2016; 409-418.

Swedo SE, Leonard HL, Rapoport JL, Lenane MC, Goldberger EL, Cheslow DL. A double blind comparison of clomipramine and desipramine in the treatment of trichotillomania. (Contains National Institute of Mental Health Trichotillomania Scales) *NEJM* 1989; 321: 497-501.

Szekely A, Kovacs-Nagy R, Banyai EI, Gosi-Greguss AC, Varga K, Halmai Z, Ronai Z, Sasvari-Szekely M. Association between hypnotizability and the catechol-o-methyltransferase (COMT) polymorphism. *Int J Clin Exper Hypn.* 2010; 58(3): 301-315.

Toledo EL, De Togni Muniz E, Brith AM, de Abreau CN, Tavares H. Group treatment for trichotillomania: cognitive-behavioral therapy versus supportive therapy. *J Clin Psychiatry* 2015: 76(4): 447-455.

Weidt S, Klaghofer R, Kuenburg A, Bruehl AB, Delsignore A, Moritz S, Rufer M. Internet-based self-help for trichotillomania: a randomized controlled study comparing decoupling and progressive muscle relaxation. *Psychother Psychosom.* 2015; 84(6):359-67.

Welch SS, Kim J. DBT-enhanced cognitive behavioral therapy for adolescent trichotillomania. *Cogn. Behav. Practice* 2012; 19: 483-493.

Winchel RM, Jones JS, Molcho A, Parsons B, Stanley B, Stanley M. The psychiatric institute trichotillomania scale (PITS). *Psychopharmacol. Bull.* 1992; 28: 463-476.

Woods DW, Wetterneck CT, Flessner CA. A controlled evaluation of acceptance and commitment therapy plus habit reversal for trichotillomania. *Behav Res Ther.* 2006; 44:639–656.

Zalsman G, Haggai Hermesh H, Sever J. Hypnotherapy in adolescents with trichotillomania: three cases, *Am J Clin Hypn* 2001; 44:1, 63-68.

In: Trichotillomania (Hair Pulling Disorder) ISBN: 978-1-53610-854-5
Editors: K. França and M. Jafferany © 2017 Nova Science Publishers, Inc.

*Chapter 7*

# TRICHOTILLOMANIA AND THE EMOTION REGULATION HYPOTHESIS

## *Erin E. Curley, BA and Nancy J. Keuthen, PhD*
Department of Psychiatry,
Massachusetts General Hospital/Harvard Medical School,
Boston, MA, US

### ABSTRACT

Emotion regulation, a transdiagnostic factor, is a burgeoning field in the study of psychopathology (Fernandez et al., 2016). Emotion regulation is broadly defined as the processes involved in and the ability to modulating emotions—specifically, maintaining positive emotions and improving negative emotions (Aparicio et al., 2016). Deficits in emotion regulation have been posited as risk factors for a variety of disorders, such as depression and anxiety (e.g., Spasojevic and Alloy, 2001).

Trichotillomania (TTM) researchers have invoked emotion regulation as one explanatory hypothesis for TTM. The emotion regulation model of TTM posits that individuals with TTM may have difficulty managing certain negative emotions and engage in hair pulling behaviors as a coping mechanism, thus relieving the negative emotional state and reinforcing the hair pulling behavior (see Roberts et al., 2013 for a recent review).

Several studies have provided empirical support for the emotion regulation hypothesis of TTM. A seminal study established the relationship between negative emotional states and TTM. In this study,

Christenson and colleagues (1993) found that negative affect and situations where negative affect might be expected (i.e., an argument) served as cues for hair pulling behavior. This research has been further corroborated in studies examining how emotional states change during the course of a hair pulling episode (e.g., Diefenbach et al., 2008). Recently, two studies have explored the ability to regulate or manage negative emotions in individuals with TTM. Shusterman and colleagues (2009) found that self-identified hair pullers had a harder time "snapping out" of negative emotional states than non-pullers. Similarly, in a second study, hair pullers had more difficulty controlling their inwardly directed anger (Curley et al., 2016). Additionally, both inability to "snap out" of negative emotional states and difficulty controlling inwardly directed anger were correlated with hair pulling severity.

Treatment studies have also provided evidence for the emotion regulation hypothesis of TTM. For example, Habit Reversal Therapy (HRT), when augmented with Dialectical Behavior Therapy, which incorporates emotion regulation strategies, effectively reduced TTM severity and impairment (Keuthen et al., 2010, 2011, 2012). Additionally, research suggests that HRT augmented with Acceptance and Commitment Therapy, which focuses on increasing the ability to tolerate the discomfort that accompanies negative emotional states, is also useful in treating TTM (Woods et al., 2006).

To further support the emotion regulation hypothesis of TTM and facilitate the creation of efficacious treatments, future research should examine whether the neuropathways and genes that have been implicated in emotion regulation deficits are also involved in TTM.

## OVERVIEW OF EMOTION

Emotion is a word that is used in everyday conversation, as well as medical and scientific discourse. As a result of the term bridging these different spheres, the definition and understanding of "emotion" is often blurred. To further complicate the matter, early theorists struggled to derive a universal, agreed upon definition of emotion. Instead, researchers conceived of emotion as an archetype and worked to outline three key features (e.g., Gross, 2008)—(1) emotions arise when an individual encounters a situation and interprets it as being relevant to their goals (Lazarus, 1991); (2) emotions are composed of related changes in the domains of subjective experience, behavior, and physiology (Mauss et al., 2005); (3) emotions are malleable and must compete with other responses triggered by the situation (James, 1884).

These three core aspects of emotions have been assembled to form a "modal model" of emotion (Barrett et al., 2007). This model dictates that "emotions arise in the context of a person-situation transaction that compels attention, has a particular meaning to an individual, and gives rise to a coordinated yet malleable multisystem response to the ongoing person-situation transaction" (Gross, 2008, pg. 499).

In addition to this overarching model of emotion, researchers have also sought to identify and classify individual emotions. Paul Ekman, a pioneer in the study of emotions, originally argued that there were six different emotions: fear, anger, surprise, happiness, and sadness (Ekman and Frisen, 19721). He argued that these six emotions were universal throughout human cultures and expanded his list to include seven additional universal emotions: embarrassment, excitement, contempt, shame, pride, satisfaction, and amusement (Ekman, 1999).

The recognition of the modal model of emotions and the early work in identifying core emotions provided the groundwork for theoretical and empirical advances in the field of emotion research. Today, there even exists a relatively accepted definition for emotion—"a complex psychological state that involves three distinct components: a subjective experience, a physiological response, and a behavioral or expressive response" (Hockenbury and Hockenbury, 2007). As researchers have gained a better understanding of emotions and have acquired more empirical knowledge on the topic, they have also begun to investigate how individuals regulate these emotions.

## EMOTION REGULATION

The first widely accepted definition of emotion regulation was offered by Ross Thompson, who wrote, "Emotion regulation consists of the extrinsic and intrinsic processes responsible for monitoring, evaluating, and modifying emotional reactions, especially their intensive and temporal features, to accomplish one's goals" (Thompson, 1994, pg. 27). Today, emotion regulation is broadly recognized as the ability and processes involved in modulating emotions—specifically, maintaining positive emotions and improving negative emotions (Aparicio et al., 2016). Deficits in emotion regulation, therefore, include the use of impulsive and harmful behaviors to modulate intense emotional experiences (Gratz and Roemer, 2004).

Emotion regulation research, although originating in developmental psychology (Gaensbauer, 1982) and often considered under the umbrella of self-regulation, has burgeoned into an independent domain inclusive of affect regulation, emotional reactivity, temperament, stress reactivity, and positive and negative emotionality. Additionally, research examining emotion regulation spans a range of psychological fields, disorders, and ages. The general consensus based on the research traversing independent fields of psychology is that the ability to regulate emotions is a broad protective factor. In regards to depression, there is an expanding body of research documenting the link between deficits in emotion regulation and the development and maintenance of depressive symptoms. For example, correlation research has demonstrated that females with major depressive disorder report greater emotion regulation difficulties compared to healthy controls (Brockmeyer et al., 2012) and prospective research suggests that differences in emotion regulation strategies predicted recovery status among depressed individuals (Arditte and Joormann, 2011). Similar relationships have also been documented between emotion regulation and other disorders, such as anxiety, substance use disorders, and eating disorders (Aldao et al., 2010). Due to the likely role of emotion regulation as a risk factor for many disorders, researchers have identified it as a transdiagnostic factor within psychopathology (Fernandez et al., 2016).

## EMOTION REGULATION HYPOTHESIS IN TRICHOTILLOMANIA

Although there has been a growing interest in trichotillomania (TTM) in the past decade, there is still a void in the research pertaining to the etiology and maintenance of this obsessive-compulsive spectrum disorder. Some researchers have suggested that emotion regulation may play a prominent role in the etiology and maintenance of TTM (see Roberts et al., 2015 for a recent review). Proponents of this theoretical model have outlined the emotion regulation hypothesis of TTM. This hypothesis posits that individuals with TTM may have deficits in emotion regulation, which cause them to have difficulties managing certain negative emotions. These individuals may engage in hair pulling as a coping mechanism, a behavior which creates a pleasurable experience or reduces the negative emotional affect. Due to these positive benefits, overtime the hair pulling behavior becomes reinforced as a coping mechanism and the TTM is maintained. A recent body of work has recently provided empirical support for this hypothesis.

# EVIDENCE OF EMOTION REGULATION IN TRICHOTILLOMANIA

## Emotional Correlates

Early studies have provided support for the emotion regulation hypothesis in TTM by establishing the link between negative emotional states and TTM. For example, in a study of seventy-five individuals with a primary diagnosis of *DSM-III-R* TTM, negative emotional states and situations involving negative affect or low self-esteem served as cues for hair pulling behavior (Christenson et al., 1993). Specifically, individuals with TTM reported pulling their hair in the context of emotions, such as embarrassment, anger, hurt, and depression; and in the context of situations, such as looking in a mirror, weighing yourself, going to the doctors, and arguments (Christenson et al., 1993). Furthermore, individuals who were more likely to pull their hair in the context of negative affective states were also more likely to endorse 'focused' hair pulling, or hair pulling that occurs within the individual's awareness (Christenson et al., 1993). Taken together, the findings of study suggest that some individuals with TTM may actively and deliberately pull their hair in response to negative emotions, thus providing rudimentary support for the emotion regulation hypothesis of TTM.

## Emotional Arcs

Building upon the evidence of emotional correlates in TTM, researchers have extended these findings by demonstrating how emotions change over the course of a pulling episode. In a study examining 44 individuals with TTM, Diefenbach and colleagues (2002) examined how emotional experiences changed throughout the course (i.e., before, during, and after) of a hair pulling episode. Results of this study demonstrated that across the episode there were significant decreases in boredom, anxiety, and tension and significant increases in guilt, relief, sadness, and anger (Diefenbach et al., 2002). The decrease in anxiety and tension and the increase in relief are compatible with the emotion regulation hypothesis of TTM. Thus, the act of hair pulling may serve to reduce negative emotional states and increase positive emotional states. It is important to note that the increases in guilt, sadness, and anger over the course of a pulling episode do not necessarily contradict the emotion regulation hypothesis of TTM. Rather, the increases in these negative emotions are likely related to the shame that many individuals with TTM feel about their hair pulling behaviors.

Subsequently, in a later study Diefenbach and colleagues (2008) examined how the changes in emotions differed between individuals with TTM and individuals without TTM. In the comparison of thirty-four participants diagnosed with TTM and thirty-two healthy volunteers, researchers found that the reported changes in emotions during the course of a hair pulling episode differed between groups (Diefenbach et al., 2006). Participants with TTM were instructed to rate 10 emotions for how they feel "before," "while," and "after" a hair pulling episode. Similarly, healthy volunteers rated the same 10 emotions for how they felt "before," while," and "after" pulling a hair for grooming purposes (Diefenbach et al., 2008). Researchers found that, while pulling, individuals with TTM reported larger decreases in boredom, tension, sadness, and anger and larger increases in relief and calm compared to healthy volunteers (Diefenbach et al., 2008). Similar to the results of the earlier study by Diefenbach and colleagues, the emotional pattern demonstrated in this study provides evidence for the emotion regulation hypothesis of TTM.

## Measures of Emotional Control

Despite the evidence based on emotional correlates and arcs in emotions for the role of emotion regulation in TTM, these earlier studies did not directly evaluate the emotion regulation hypothesis of TTM. In an online study examining 1162 self-reported hair pullers and 175 controls, Shusterman and colleagues (2009) aimed to investigate three specific aspects of the emotion regulation hypothesis of TTM: (1) do hair pullers have greater difficulty modulating their emotions than controls?, (2) do pullers with greater difficulty regulating their emotions have greater hair pulling severity?, and (3) are the emotions that individual hair pullers have difficulty regulating more likely to be a trigger for a pulling episode? The results of the study support each of the three aspects of the emotion regulation hypothesis of TTM that Shusterman examined. First, the results of the study suggested that individuals with TTM experienced more difficulty modulating their emotions compared to non-pullers. Second, the degree of emotional control and regulation was correlated with hair-pulling severity—specifically, that individuals who have more difficulty "snapping out" of negative emotions also had more severe hair pulling. Finally, the researchers found that the level of difficulty regulating certain emotions is predictive of the degree to which those emotions trigger hair pulling episodes. Thus, the findings of this internet study establish that there is an evident link between emotion regulation and TTM.

One of the most recent studies to provide evidence supporting the emotion regulation hypothesis of TTM built upon these internet findings. A study was conducted examining the association between anger and hair pulling in a sample of 158 women with diagnosed chronic hair pulling disorder (met *DSM-IV-TR* TTM diagnosis except for tension and/or relief criteria) or *DSM-IV-TR* TTM (Curley et al., 2016). Interestingly, when compared to an age and gender matched normative population, individuals with TTM did not differ on trait anger, suggesting that they do not have a particular proneness to experiencing anger as a general tendency or when provoked. However, when they were to experience anger, individuals with TTM were more likely than the normative sample to experience inwardly directed anger and they had a harder time controlling or reducing this inward anger. That individuals with TTM are more likely to experience inwardly directed anger and have difficulty managing this anger suggests that hair pullers may have trouble regulating their anger—supporting the emotion regulation model of TTM. In other words, certain individuals who have trouble regulating emotions, such as anger, may attend to these emotional situations by engaging in hair pulling behaviors as a coping mechanism.

Further supporting the emotion regulation model of TTM, Curley and colleagues (2016) found that the frequency with which individuals with TTM reported experiencing inwardly directed anger was significantly correlated with hair pulling severity. Beyond that, the frequency of inwardly directed anger predicted hair pulling severity above and beyond levels of depression and anxiety. These findings fit within the theory of emotion and the emotion regulation model—an individual with TTM encounters a situation, which they attend to, and thus experience inwardly directed anger. To regulate these unwanted emotions, the individual turns to hair pulling to reduce the discomfort, as this behavior becomes conditioned, the individual engages in more frequent hair pulling to modulate anger, and therefore has more severe hair pulling.

## TREATMENT IMPLICATIONS

The extant body of literature on the emotion regulation hypothesis of TTM supports the position that emotion regulation plays a role in TTM. Due to the relationship between emotion regulation and TTM, it may be beneficial for the treatment of TTM to teach adaptive coping strategies and alternative techniques for regulating emotions. Currently, the gold standard treatment is Habit Reversal Training (HRT); a branch of cognitive-behavior therapy (CBT) designed to treat repetitive behaviors (Azrin and Nunn, 1973, Azrin et al., 1980). There are three main components involved in HRT: (1) awareness training to help patients recognize the triggers of their hair pulling, (2) competing response training to teach patients to substitute the pulling with alternative, incompatible behaviors (i.e., creating a fist), and (3) social support training to help the patient maintain the treatment strategies (Azrin and Nunn, 1973, Azrin et al., 1980). However, this standardized HRT protocol fails to address the intense emotions that are often related to hair pulling behavior (e.g., Flessner et al., 2008, Keuthen et al., 2010, Woods, et al., 2006). To date, two studies have explored augmenting this traditional treatment with protocols that target emotion regulation and experiential avoidance.

## Treatment Augmentation with Acceptance and Commitment Therapy

The first study tested Acceptance and Commitment Therapy (ACT) enhanced HRT (Woods et al., 2006). ACT is a process-based approach targeting experiential avoidance (Hayes et al., 1999). Experiential avoidance is a coping strategy in which an individual is unwilling to experience certain (often negative) feelings, physiological sensations, and thoughts, and thus attempts to alter the form or frequency of these experiences (Hayes et al., 1996). Experiential avoidance is addressed within the ACT protocol by using acceptance and mindfulness to decrease maladaptive emotion regulation and produce behavioral change within the client (Hayes et al., 1999).

When applied to TTM, the ACT protocol functions to create a context where individuals can experience and accept urges to engage in hair pulling behavior, but not engage in the behavior (Crosby et al., 2012). Therefore, from an emotion regulation perspective, ACT could teach individuals with TTM to experience and accept the emotional triggers that may trigger them to pull their hair, rather than engaging in negative coping mechanisms.

Woods and colleagues (2006) found that HRT augmented with CBT is an effective treatment. After ten sessions of ACT enhanced HRT, individuals showed improvement in their TTM symptoms, less experiential avoidance, and reduced depressive and anxiety symptoms compared to their pre-treatment scores and versus the waitlist control group. Specifically, individuals who received the augmented treatment demonstrated reductions in hair pulling severity, hair pulling impairment, number of pulled hairs, experiential avoidance scores, and anxiety and depressive symptom. Furthermore, the majority of these improvements were maintained through the 3-month follow-up. These findings demonstrate that addressing the emotional triggers of hair pulling and physical sensations involved in experiential avoidance may be an effective augmentation of the standard gold treatment of TTM.

## Treatment Augmentation with Dialectical Behavior Therapy

The second study examined the efficacy of HRT augmented with Dialectical Behavioral Therapy (DBT) techniques in reducing hair pulling severity and impairment (Keuthen et al., 2010, 2011, 2012). The primary theoretical aim of the DBT approach is to help individuals improve their emotional and cognitive regulation skills (Linehan 1993a, 1993b). Unlike ACT, which is conceptually abstract and is not centered around the delivery of skills, the aims of DBT are accomplished by the utilization of four primary skill sets—mindfulness, distress tolerance, interpersonal effectiveness, and emotion regulation (Linehan 1993a, 1993b). In other words, DBT helps the individual learn about the triggers that lead to reactive states and teaches them to adaptively assess which coping skills to apply in order to avoid or reduce the unwanted or undesired situation. DBT has been shown to be effective in treating other disorders that are characterized by affective dysregulation and impulsivity (i.e., substance dependence and eating disorders).

Based on the emotion regulation hypothesis of TTM, there is evidence to believe that DBT would also be an effective treatment for individuals with TTM. DBT for TTM would target the emotional triggers that cause the individual to engage in hair pulling as a coping mechanism and would then teach more adaptive skills to modulate these emotions.

Keuthen and colleagues (2011) demonstrated that HRT augmented with DBT was an effective treatment for individuals with TTM. After eleven sessions of treatment, the individuals in the treatment group receiving the augmented therapy displayed significant improvement in TTM severity and impairment, experiential avoidance, and mood and anxiety symptoms. Furthermore, these individuals showed significant gains in their emotion regulation skills. Three- and sixth-month follow-up suggests that these improvements, particularly improvements in emotion regulation, are maintained after the active therapy has finished (Keuthen et al., 2012). Taken together, this preliminary study of DBT augmented treatment for TTM establishes that addressing emotion regulation capabilities is an important aspect of TTM treatment and augmented treatment is an effective way to target these deficits.

## FUTURE RESEARCH

As a fairly new topic in psychopathology research, studies investigating all components of the emotional regulation hypothesis of TTM are warranted and needed. Specifically, following the direction of the current psychology field, research exploring the emotional regulation hypothesis of TTM from a biological psychology approach may be particularly relevant. In recent years, both genetics and neural correlates have become crucial for understanding the link between emotion regulation and psychopathology.

### Genetics

Research examining the genetics of emotion regulation started broadly with the question of heritability. Early studies provided heritability estimates of 40-50% for emotion-related personality traits (i.e., neuroticism and extraversion), which provided early evidence for the role of genetics in the individual differences in reaction and response to emotional stimuli (Viken et al., 1994, Jang et al., 1996). Extending this initial evidence for heritability, Soussignan and colleagues (2009) conducted a twin study with five-month-old twin pairs and found evidence for heritability in emotion regulation based on their gaze aversion to strangers' facial expressions. The very limited heritability research that is available provides preliminary support for the idea that differences in emotion regulation are, in part, genetically moderated.

Building upon this, genetics studies have identified possible molecular genetic associations of emotion regulation. Currently, three candidate gene polymorphisms are being considered in the genetic moderation of emotion regulation. The first polymorphism, a single nucleotide polymorphism on the serotonin transporter gene (5-HTTLPR) has been associated with increased activation in brain regions (e.g., the amygdala) involved in emotional processing (Hariri et al., 2002, Canli et al., 2005, Hermann et al., 2007, Munafo et al., 2008). Another polymorphism, Catechol-o-Methyltransferase

(COMT) Val[158]Met, has been implicated in moderating the frontal cortical involvement in top-down emotion regulation (Chen et al., 2004). This polymorphism has been demonstrated to be involved in COMT (an enzyme that degrades catecholamines) activity, which affects the dopamine catabolism in the prefrontal cortex (Chen et al., 2004). Therefore, individuals with the risk alleles on this polymorphism may have greater levels of dopamine in their prefrontal cortex, which may cause deficits in emotion regulation (Chen et al., 2004). The final polymorphism, monoamine oxidase A, has also been linked to brain circuits involved in emotion and emotion regulation (Buckholtz et al., 2008, Buckholtz and Meyer-Lindenberg, 2008).

Albeit very preliminary, there exists both heritability research and genetic association research suggesting that emotion regulation, at least in part, may be linked to or moderated by genetics. Future TTM research should examine whether these identified genes have any influence on the development of TTM.

## Neural Correlates

Studies examining the neural correlates of emotion regulation are even sparser. However, there is research suggesting that there are multiple brain regions that are involved in emotions—all cortical lobes, subcortical structures, and the cerebellum (Phan, et al., 2002, Pullips et al., 2003). Specifically, the dorsomedial prefrontal cortex is involved in multiple components of emotion regulation (Amodio and Frith, 2006. Oschner et al., 2014), the ventromedial prefrontal cortex and the orbitofrontal cortex are involved in determining outcomes and goals (Kringelbach, 2005, Berns et al., 2001), and the amygdala is responsible for generating emotional responses (Vuillemier, 2005). Researchers should work to examine whether there are differences in these brain regions and structures among individuals with and without TTM.

## CONCLUSION

It is evident from the extant body of literature that emotion regulation is a transdiagnostic factor implicated in TTM. The current emotion regulation hypothesis of TTM suggests that individuals with TTM may have deficits in emotion regulation skills and therefore engage in hair pulling to reduce negative affective states. While the previous literature provides a strong empirical foundation for the emotion regulation hypothesis of TTM, future research is needed. First, researchers should seek to replicate and illuminate past research exploring the phenomenological characteristics of emotion regulation in TTM. Second, only two studies have examined outcomes of treatment targeting emotion regulation deficits. Additional treatment outcome studies exploring protocols that address emotion regulation are needed to determine the effectiveness of these types of treatments. Finally, researchers should extend investigations examining the aforementioned polymorphisms and neural correlates in a TTM population, as well as explore additional genetic and neurologic factors. In examining these three aims, we will be able to gain a better understanding of TTM, emotion regulation, and the relationship between the two.

## REFERENCES

Aldao A., Nolen-Hoeksema S. and Schweizer S. (2010). Emotion-regulation strategies across psychopathology: A meta-analytic review. *Clinical Psychology Review, 30*(2), 217-237.

Amodio DM. and Frith CD. (2006). Meeting of minds: the medial frontal cortex and social cognition. Nature Reviews Neuroscience, 7(4), 268-277.

Aparicio E., Canals J., Arija V., De Hemauw S. and Michels N. (2016). The role of emotion regulation in childhood obesity: implications for prevention and treatment. *Nutrition Research Reviews* doi:10.1017/ S0954422415000153.

Arditte KA. and Joormann J. (2011). Emotion regulation in depression: reflection predicts recovery from a major depressive episode. *Cognitive Therapy and Research, 35*(6), 536-543.

Azrin NH. and Nunn RG. (1973). Habit-reversal: A method for eliminating nervous habits and tics. *Behaviour Research and Therapy, 11*, 619-628.

Azrin NH., Nunn RG. and Frantz SE. (1980). Treatment of hairpulling (trichotillomania): A comparative study of habit reversal and negative practice training. *Journal of Behavior Therapy and Experimental Psychiatry, 11*, 13-20.

Barrett LF., Ochsner KN. and Gross JJ (2007). On the automaticity of emotion. In J. Bargh (Ed.) *Social psychology and the unconscious: The automaticity of higher mental processes.* New York: Psychology Press.

Berns GS., McClure SM., Pagnoni G. and Montague PR. (2001). Predictability modulates human brain response to reward. The *Journal of Neuroscience, 21(8),* 2793-2798.

Brockmeyer T., Bents H., Groose M., Pfeiffer N., Herzog W. and Friederich, H-C. (2012). Specific emotion regulation impairments in major depression and anorexia nervosa. *Psychiatry Research, 200,* 550-553.

Buckholtz, JW., Callicott JH., Kolachana B., Hariri AR., Goldberg TE., Genderson M., Egan MF., Mattay VS., et al., (2008). Genetic variation in MAOA modulates ventromedial prefrontal circuitry mediating individual differences in human personality. *Molecular Psychiatry, 13,* 313-324.

Buckholtz JW. and Meyer-Lindenberg A. (2008). MAOA and the neruogenetic architecture of human aggression. *Trends in Neurosciences, 31,* 120-129.

Canli T., Omura K., Hass BW., Fallgatter AJ., Constable RT. and Lesch K. (2005). Beyond affect: A role for genetic variation of the serotonin transporter in neural activation during a cognitive attention task. *Proceedings of the National Academy of Science, 102,* 12224-12229.

Chen J., Lipska BK., Halim N., Ma QD., Matsumoto M., Melhem S., Kolachana BS., Hyde TM., Hermann MN et al., (2004). Functional analysis of genetic variation in catechol-O-methyltransferase (COMT): Effects on mRNA, protein, and enzyme activity in postmortem human brain. *Journal of Human Genetics, 75,* 807-821.

Christenson GA., Ristvedt SL. and MacKenzie TB. (1993). Identification of trichotillomania cue profiles. *Behavior Research and Therapy 31*(3), 315-320.

Crosby JM., Dehlin JP., Mithcell PR. and Twohig MP. (2012). Acceptance and commitment therapy and habit reversal training for the treatment of trichotillomania. *Cognitive and Behavioral Practice, 19,* 595-605.

Diefenbach GJ., Tolin DF, Meuier SK. and Worhunsky P. (2008). Emotion regulation and trichotillomania: a comparison of clinical and nonclinical hair pulling. *Journal of Behavior Therapy and Experimental Psychiatry, 39*(1), 32-14.

Ekman P. and Frisen WV. (1971). Constants across cultures in the face and emotion. *Journal of Personality and Social Psychology, 17,* 124-129.

Ekman P. (1999). Basic emotions. In T. Dalgleish and Power, M (Ed.) *Handbook of Cognition and Emotion.* Sussex, UK: John Wiley and Sons.

Fernandez KC., Jaxaieri H. and Gross JJ. (2016). Emotion regulation: a transdiagnostic perspective on a new RDoc domain. *Cogn Ther Res* doi: 10.1007/s10608-016-9772-2.

Flessner CA., Conelea CA., Woods DW., Franklin ME. and Keuthen NJ. (2008). Styles of pulling in trichotillomania: Exploring differences in symptom severity, phenomenology, and functional impairment. *Behaviour Research and Therapy, 46*, 345-357.

Gaensbauer TJ. (1982). Regulation of emotional expression in infants from two contrasting caretaking environments. *Journal of American Academy of Child Psychiatry, 21*, 163-170.

Gratz KL and Roemer L. (2003). Multidimensional assessment of emotion regulation and dysregulation: Development, factor structure, and initial validation of the Difficulties in Emotion Regulation Scale. *Journal of Psychopathology and Behavioral Assessment, 26*(1), 41-54.

Hariri AR., Mattay VS., Tessitore A., Kolachana B., Fera F., Goldman D., Egan MF. and Weinberger DR. (2002). Serotonin transporter genetic variation and the response of the human amygdala. *Science, 297*, 400-403.

Hayes SC., Strosahl KD. and Wilson KG. (1999). *Acceptance and commitment therapy: An experiential approach to behavior change.* New York: Guilford Press.

Hayes SC., Wilson KG., Gifford EV., Follette VM. and Strosahl KD. (1996). Experiential avoidance and behavior disorders: A functional dimensional approach to diagnosis and treatment. *Journal of Consulting and Clinical Psychology, 64*, 1152-1168.

Hermann MJ., Huter T., Muller F., Muhlberger A., Pauli P., Reif A., Renner T., Canli T., Fallgatter AJ. and Lesch KP. (2007). Additive effects of serotonin transporter and trytophan hydroxylase-2 gene variation on emotional processing. *Cerebral Cortex, 17,* 1160-1163.

Hockenbury DH. and Hockenbury SE. (2007). *Discovering psychology.* New York: Worth Publishers.

James W. (1884). What is an emotion? *Mind, 9,* 188-205.

Jang KL., Livesley WJ. and Vernon PA. Heritability of the big five personality dimensions and their facets: A twin study. *Journal of Personality, 64,* 577-591.

Keuthen NJ., Flessner CA., Woods DW., Franklin ME., Stein DJ. and Cashin SE., (2007). Factor Analysis of the Massachusetts General Hospital Hair Pulling Scale. *Journal of Psychosomatic Research 62*(6), 707-709.

Keuthen NJ., Rothbaum BO., Falkenstein BA., Meunier S., Timpano KR., Jenike MA., et al., (2011). DBT-enhanced habit reversal treatment for trichotillomania: 3- and 6-month follow-up results. *Depression and Anxiety, 28*(4), 310-313.

Keuthen NJ., Rothbaum BO., Fama J., Altenburger E., Falkenstein MJ., Sprich SE., et al., (2012). DBT-enhanced habit reversal treatment for trichotillomania: A randomized controlled trial. *Journal of Behavioral Addictions, 1*(3), 1-9.

Keuthen NJ., Rothbaum BO., Welch SS., Taylor C., Falkenstein M., Heekin M., et al., (2010). Pilot trial of dialectical behavior therapy-enhanced habit reversal for trichotillomania. *Depression and Anxiety, 27*(10), 953-959.

Kringelbach ML. (2005). The human orbitofrontal cortex: linking reward to hedonic experience. *Nature Reviews Neuroscience, 6(9)*, 691-702.

Lazarus R. S. (1991). *Emotion and adaptation.* Oxford: Oxford University Press.

Linehan MM. (1993a). *Cognitive-behavioral Treatment of Borderline Personality Disorder.* New York: Guilford Press.

Linehan MM (1993b). *Skills Training Manual for Treating Borderline Personality Disorder.* New York: Guilford Press.

Mauss IB., Levenson RW., McCarter L., Wihelm FH. and Gross JJ. (2005). The tie that bind?: Coherence among emotion experience, behavior, and physiology. *Emotions, 5,* 175-190.

Mufano MR., Brown SM. and Hariri AR. (2008). Serotonin transporter (5-HTTLPR) genotype and amygdala activation: a meta-analysis. *Biological Psychiatry, 63,* 852-857.

Ochsner KN., Knierim K., Ludlow DH., Hanelin J., Ramachandran T., Glover G. and Mackey SC. (2004). Reflecting upon feelings: an fMRI study of neural systems supporting the attribution of emotion to self and other. *Journal of Cognitive Neuroscience, 16(10),* 1746-1772.

Phan KL., Wager T., Taylor S F. and Liberzon I. (2002). Functional neuroanatomy of emotion: a meta-analysis of emotion activation studies in PET and fMRI. *Neuroimage, 16*(2), 331-348.

Phillips ML., Drevets WC., Rauch SL. and Lane R. (2003). Neurobiology of emotion perception I: The neural basis of normal emotion perception. *Biological Psychiatry, 54(5),* 504-514.

Roberts S., O'Connor K. and Belanger C. (2013). Emotion regulation and other psychological models for body-focused repetitive behaviors. *Clinical Psychology Review, 33*(6), 651-662.

Soussignan R., Boivin M., Girad A., Perusse D., Liu X. and Tremblay RE. (2009). Genetic and environmental etiology of emotional and social behaviors in 5-month-old infant twins: Influence of the social context. *Infant Behavior and Development, 32,* 1-9.

Spasojevic J. and Alloy LB. (2001). Rumination as a common mechanism relating depressive risk factors to depression. *Emotion, 1*(1), 25-37.

Thompson, RA. (1994). Development of emotion regulation: biological and behavioral considerations. *Monographs of the Society for Research in Child Development, 59,* 25-52.

Viken RJ., Rose RH., Kaprio J.,& Koshenvuo M. (1994). A developmental genetic analysis of adult personality: Extraversion and neuroticism from 18 to 59 years of age. *Journal of Personality and Social Psychology, 66,* 722-730/

Vuilleumier P. (2005). How brains beware: neural mechanisms of emotional attention. *Trends in Cognitive Sciences, 9(12),* 585-594.

Woods DW., Wetterneck CT. and Flessner CA (2006). A controlled evaluation of acceptance and commitment therapy plus habit reversal for trichotillomania. *Behavior Research and Therapy, 44*(5), 639-656.

# Index

## A

acceptance and commitment therapy, 75, 78, 83, 84, 86, 92, 97, 98, 100
addictive, 13, 14
affect regulation, 24, 88
Alopecia Areata, 36, 37, 38, 40, 41, 42, 45, 46, 49, 50, 51, 52
ancient Greek, 2
androgenetic Alopecia, 15, 38, 42, 46, 51
antipsychotics, 28, 56, 65, 66
anxiety, 9, 11, 12, 13, 14, 18, 21, 23, 29, 30, 31, 49, 56, 68, 76, 79, 80, 85, 88, 89, 91, 92, 93, 98, 99
anxiety disorder, 23
anxiolytics, 28
assessment tools, 26, 27
automatic/habitual type, 19
Axis I comorbidity, 23, 32

## B

behavioral models, 23, 25
biologic, 23
blepharitis, 26
body dysmorphic disorder, 6, 19, 22, 32
body-focused repetitive behavior, 13, 14
body-focused repetitive behavior disorders, 13, 14
brain abnormalities, 24

## C

cannabinoid agonist, 28, 34, 59, 69
capsaicin, 28
childhood, 24
childhood onset, 18
childhood trauma, 24
classic Pseudopelade of Brocq, 38, 39, 50
cognitive factors, 20
cognitive-behavioral therapy, 67, 75, 77, 78, 83
comorbidities, 6, 14, 23, 26
competing response procedures, 28
congenital temporal triangular alopecia, 38, 39, 47
coping strategies, 12, 28, 92
cortical thickness, 24, 33

## D

depression, 3, 9, 11, 12, 14, 21, 23, 29, 30, 49, 56, 57, 59, 70, 78, 79, 85, 88, 89, 91, 96, 97, 98, 99, 100
dermatopathology, vii, ix, 35, 36, 52
diagnostic and statistical manual of mental disorders, 5, 7
dialectic behavioral therapy, 75
differential diagnoses, 22, 35, 36, 37, 38, 40, 41, 42, 47, 49, 50, 51
diffusion tensor imaging, 24, 33

disorder, 1, 6, 22, 23, 25, 29, 32, 33, 57, 59, 63, 64, 65, 66, 71, 72, 73, 76
Dronabinol, 28, 29, 34, 69

## E

emotion regulation, ix, 85, 86, 87, 88, 89, 90, 91, 92, 93, 94, 95, 96, 97, 98, 99, 100
emotional aspects, 11
epidemiology, 18

## F

familial, 6, 19, 31
Fiddling sheep, 18
focused/compulsive type, 19
functional neuroimaging, 24

## G

genetic, 8, 24, 25, 79, 94, 95, 96, 97, 98, 99, 100
genetic factors, 8, 24
glutamatergic agents, 28

## H

habit reversal therapy, 22, 27, 28, 29, 57
habit reversal training, 75, 77, 92, 97
hair, ix, 11, 12, 14, 22, 49
hair disorder, ix, 11, 12, 14, 22, 49
hair pulling, 2, 3, 4, 5, 6, 7, 9, 13, 15, 17, 18, 19, 21, 22, 23, 24, 25, 27, 28, 30, 31, 32, 33, 34, 56, 58, 61, 64, 66, 67, 68, 69, 75, 76, 77, 79, 80, 81, 85, 86, 88, 89, 90, 91, 92, 93, 95, 97
hair pulling disorder, i, iii, 1, 2, 6, 7, 9, 13, 15, 17, 33, 68, 91
histopathological findings, 26, 35, 36, 37, 41, 48
history, vii, 1, 2, 8, 9, 14, 15, 19, 24, 29, 31, 36, 47, 53, 80
Hoxb8, 25, 33

hypnoanalysis with ideomotor signaling, 81
hypnosis, 80, 82, 83
hypnotic suggestion, 75, 80
hypochondriasis, 19

## I

impulse control disorder, 6, 30, 76

## L

lithium, 28, 59, 69

## M

management, ix, xi, 9, 14, 29, 63, 65, 66, 102
Massachusetts General Hospital Hair Pulling Scale, 62, 77, 98
mental health, 13
milk thistle, 56, 65, 73
modeling theory, 25
motivation enhancement, 28
motor habits, 24
motor tic, 19
movement decoupling, 78, 83
MRI findings, 23
myo-inositol, 56, 65, 67

## N

$N$-Acetylcysteine [NAC], 28, 29, 34, 56, 59, 60, 61, 62, 63, 64, 65, 66, 67, 70, 71, 72
nail biting, 18, 22, 64, 65, 72, 76
naltrexone, 28, 58, 68
National Institute of Mental Health, 78, 83
National Institute of Mental Health Trichotillomania Scales, 78, 83
neuroanatomical studies, 24
neurobiology, 24, 32, 71, 99
non-rapid eye movement (NREM), 20, 31
nucleus accumbens, 24
nutraceuticals, 56, 66, 73

# Index

## O

object relation theory, 24
obsessive compulsive disorder (OCD), 1, 6, 22, 23, 25, 29, 32, 33, 57, 59, 63, 64, 65, 66, 71, 72, 73, 76
obsessive-compulsive related disorders, 56, 67
Olanzapine, 28, 34, 58, 68

## P

pathophysiology, 23, 71
personality traits, 21, 32, 94
pharmacological treatment, ix, 27, 55, 56, 75, 76
pigment casts, 26, 35, 42, 43, 44, 45, 47, 48, 49, 51
post-traumatic stress disorder, 19
premenstrual, 20
pressure Alopecia, 35, 38, 47, 51
prevalence, 18, 30, 31
prognosis, 26, 53
psychiatric comorbidity, 23, 30
Psychiatric Institute Trichotillomania Scale, 27, 62, 78, 84
psychoanalysis, 75, 76, 77
psychoanalytical, 23
psychodermatology, xi, 2, 8, 12, 14, 49, 53, 102, 103
psychoemotional stress, 12
psychosocial dysfunction, 21
psychosomatic hypnoanalysis, 75, 81

## Q

quality of life, 12, 13, 15, 21, 31

## R

relaxation training, 28, 77
response covariation theory, 25

## S

SAPAP3, 25, 33
scales, 26, 27, 57, 77
screening, 26, 27, 40, 81
self-esteem, 12, 21, 36, 49, 89
self-monitoring, 26, 27, 28, 77
self-regulation, 88
sexual abuse, 24
Shakespeare, vii, 1, 3, 4, 8, 9
silymarin, 56, 65, 67, 73
skin picking, 9, 15, 18, 22, 31, 32, 33, 56, 64, 66, 72, 74, 83, 103
SLITRIK1, 25
somatic bridge, 81
St. John's wort, 56, 65, 66, 67
stimulus, 28, 77, 79
stimulus control, 28, 77, 79
structural abnormalities, 23, 24
substance use disorder, 23, 88
suicide attempts, 23
Syphilitic Alopecia, 37, 38, 39, 40, 50, 52

## T

tension reduction theory, 25
Tinea Capitis, 37, 38, 40, 50
topical steroids, 28
Tourette syndrome, 19
Traction Alopecia, 37, 38, 41, 47, 48, 50, 51, 52
transitional objects, 28
treatment, 15, 18, 22, 25, 26, 27, 28, 29, 30, 31, 34, 52, 55, 56, 57, 58, 59, 61, 62, 63, 64, 65, 66, 67, 68, 69, 71, 72, 73, 74, 76, 77, 78, 79, 80, 81, 82, 83, 86, 91, 92, 93, 96, 97, 98, 99
trichobezoars,, 26
trichodaganomania, 26, 34
trichomalacia, 35, 40, 42, 43, 44, 45, 47, 48, 49, 51
trichopsychodermatology, vii, 11, 12, 13, 14, 102
trichorrizophagia, 25, 34

trichoteiromania, 25, 34, 38, 41, 45, 50
trichotemnomania, 25, 34, 37, 38, 41, 50, 53
trichotillomania, i, iii, vii, ix, xi, 1, 2, 3, 5, 6, 7, 8, 9, 11, 12, 13, 14, 15, 17, 18, 19, 20, 21, 22, 23, 24, 25, 26, 27, 28, 29, 30, 31, 32, 33, 34, 35, 36, 37, 38, 39, 40, 41, 42, 43, 44, 45, 46, 47, 48, 49, 50, 51, 53, 55, 56, 59, 61, 62, 66, 67, 68, 69, 71, 72, 74, 75, 76, 77, 78, 79, 80, 81, 82, 83, 84, 85, 88, 89, 96, 97, 98, 99, 100, 103
tricyclic antidepressant, 28, 56

triggers, 18, 20, 92, 93

## U

unresolved conflict, 76

## W

White matter studies, 24